Massah and Meribah
(Exodus 17:7)

Repeated

by physicians,

and other members of the medical sciences.

Copyright © 2009 Ruth Oliver, M.B. Ch.B., F.R.C.P.(C).

All rights reserved

No part of this book may be reproduced, stored in a retrieval system, or transmitted by any means, electronic, mechanical, photocopying, recording, or otherwise, without written permission from the author or publisher. There is one exception. Brief passages may be quoted in articles or reviews.

Library and Archives Canada Cataloguing in Publication

CIP data on file with the National Library and Archives

ISBN 978-1-926582-41-2

For those interested in the actual "Words" see Some examples page 91. Book, " Medicine of God "in print shortly. ISBN 978-1-926582-43-6
Contact information :web address http://www.epistleoflove.org/
Email: info@epistleoflove.org

Some Reflections upon God and The Medical Sciences

A Warning for Physicians and Others in the Medical and paramedical Professions.
(Massah and Meribah repeated.)

In Old and New Testaments there are numerous examples of good and evil human behavior. God always responds with "a Blessing or a Curse."(Deut 28-OT. and Do not imagine that I have come to abolish the Law or the Prophets. I have come not to abolish but to complete them (*Mt 5:17-20;* The Beatitudes). Physicians embraced the "culture of death," and abandoned the Hippocratic Oath. Now most medical graduates worldwide swear no Oath upholding the sacredness of human life.

As most are aware (except patients it seems), between 30 and 40 years ago, Physicians abandoned the Hippocratic Oath. When I graduated from medical school in 1971 our tradition was that we swore the Hippocratic Oath the day after our exam results were published, before any of us started our internship. Now most medical graduates worldwide, including the medical school I graduated from, do not.

So the Hippocratic Oath, a pre-Christian symbol, has now fallen into worldwide disuse, with probably no more than two percent of medical graduates if that, still swearing the Hippocratic Oath at graduation. It surprises me how few patients that I have asked actually know that. Most patients I have asked still believe doctors swear the Hippocratic Oath. However, most physicians have a well worked out path by which we have, habitually by now, learned to show acts of mercy to our patients. But if any of you are like me, we hesitate to do anything that makes us conspicuously different before our colleagues.

However, since I believe that what matters won't change, and what changes won't matter; if one pays sufficient attention and perseveres, one is rewarded with insights on things eternal, on perennial values, including the contemplation of the mystery of God, present in everyday reality. It is hard not to notice how much moral values have deteriorated, even disappeared since the Hippocratic Oath was abandoned.

There is a consequence to me personally, for every decision I make, even if it is not always instant, but may be worked out in the long term as my life unfolds. The words of St Peter come to mind: **"But there is one thing, my friends, that you must never forget: that with the Lord, 'a day' can mean a thousand years, and** *a thousand years is like a day.* **[2P 3:8]** We are limited by time, but God the Alpha and Omega [Rv 1:8]of all time is not! **For My Ways are not your ways and My Time is not your time! [Is 55:8-9].**

Now it may seem like old news and we may not think it relevant to us in our times- that when Moses led the Israelites out of Egypt, the Israelites often doubted and frequently defected from the path chosen by God for them. They reverted to practices that were idolatrous in God's Eyes, rather than trust God and do things His Way. God therefore abandoned them wandering in the desert for forty years, till all who had rebelled had died in the desert, before leading their descendants to the Promised Land.

He allowed them to wander but not to be totally extinguished. When they had no water, He told Aaron and Moses to gather the people and strike the rock from which water would flow, and manifest God's holiness. But Moses and Aaron struck the rock twice, which God, the Reader of our hearts, saw to be an act of disbelief that God could manifest His holiness. For punishment the two were allowed to see, but not enter the promised land. [Num 20:12].

God was laying down a blueprint –a prototype of how it will always be between humankind and our Creator. As God says in **Deuteronomy 30:19-20, "I set before you life or death, blessing or curse. Choose life then so that you and your descendants may live in the love of Yahweh your God, obeying his voice, clinging to Him; for in this your life consists, and on this depends your long stay in the land which Yahweh swore to your fathers, Abraham, Isaac and Jacob He would give to them. "**

Throughout Man's history in Scripture this theme repeats itself. God has always shown, through His prophets in the Old Testament, and in the New Testament through His Son Jesus Christ and His Apostles and Disciples guided and inspired by His Holy Spirit, and their descendants continuously throughout time, what God's Will is for mankind, and how It is to be lived. As Jesus Himself told us,"**Do not imagine that I have come to abolish the Law or the Prophets. I have come not to abolish but to complete them. I tell you solemnly, till heaven and earth disappear, not one dot, not one little stroke, shall disappear from the Law, until its purpose is achieved. Therefore, the man who infringes even one of the least of these commandments and teaches others to do the same, will be considered the least in the kingdom of heaven; but the man who keeps them and teaches them will be considered great in the kingdom of heaven. For I tell you, if your virtue goes no deeper than that of the scribes and Pharisees, you will never get into the kingdom of heaven."**[*Mt 5:17-20;* The Beatitudes.]

Jesus, whose Mission on earth was and is, to teach and to heal, then proceeds, throughout the Gospels, to set an even higher standard by which we should live and will be judged. [summarized in M*t 25:31-46*].

However, from the times of Adam and Eve, God has also given us the free will to choose to obey His Will or not. I suppose it could not be otherwise. If we are to choose His Will out of love for Him, and not just out of fear, then He had to give us free will, knowing to His Sorrow, that many of us would rebel. Some of us would choose not to love Him, at whatever cost this rebellion to us. No matter how much He loved us, He had chosen not to force us to love Him.

He would only show us, through His Son, how much He loved us. As Jesus told us, **"if anyone love Me he will keep my word, and my Father will love him, and we shall come to him and make our home with him. Those who do not love me do not keep my words. And my word is not my own: it is the word of the one who sent me."[Jn 14:23-24]**. He also shows us the cost and the reward of a life of discipleship. So, measured in this His Light, how are the physicians, the healers, doing so far?

What can be confusing, is how longsuffering and patient God is! I think that as a result, some of us sometimes deceive ourselves into thinking that either God does not exist, or that He really is not concerned about the doings of humankind, or that He cannot possibly be aware of each and every little thing that each and every person does at every moment of our lives. But that is our limitation-our inability to grasp the concept of eternal, Divine omniscience, omnipresence and omnipotence; the eternal NOW!

Granted, it is impossible for us to grasp how small earth becomes when viewed from heaven! Nevertheless, we are invited to use our Faith, with all of our faculties-of sight, imagination, sound, smell, taste, touch, to grasp fully the Presence of the Divine in everything and in each moment .
I have come to understand that Jesus came, as Man through woman, exactly as we do, so there is no human experience that Jesus did not either experience or know about. Therefore He can authentically show us that there is a Way to live a human life that pleases God. As He Himself told us, **"I am the Way, the Truth and the Life. No-one comes to the Father except through Me."[Jn14:6]**. Jesus also showed us how utterly, unfailingly faithful to God He was, even unto His brutal torture and eventual Death on the Cross.

Since Jesus is the perfect man, like us in all things but sin, it makes sense to me, that He is also to be the One who opens the scroll: **"He, the Lion of the tribe of Judah, the Root of David, He Who stood between the throne with its four animals and the circle of elders, the Lamb Who seemed to have been sacrificed," [Revelation 5:4-6]**. He will open up the scroll which He takes from the right hand of the One sitting on the throne, which has seven seals which He breaks and proceeds to mete out the consequences. We will be judged according to how we have honoured God Our Creator and how we have treated fellow human beings. (Mt25:36-45). As St John says**," For the Father who is the Source of Life, has made the Son the source of Life; and, because he is the Son of Man, has appointed him supreme judge." [Jn5:26-27.]**

Here we come up against yet another of our latter-day snags. Many physicians have seemingly lost the idea of who are our fellow human beings. We seem to be constantly lost in disputes about whether the embryo, or the pre-born baby or the deformed one e.g (anencephalic) baby is, or is not, a fellow human being. The core Truth to have before our eyes at all times, is that God as the Author of Life, does not create human lives randomly. In His great Love He chooses every life and breathes His Life into each one, with a specific purpose for that human life to accomplish in His Name on this earth, in a specific time frame; the length of that life. This happens whether or not we are conscious of His Purpose here on earth for us.

Furthermore, even though mothers and fathers are the pro-creators who provide what is needed for the formation of the body of that new human being, God alone bestows Life (the soul) if He so desires and for His Purposes. As I understand it, every soul is created perfectly, in the image and likeness of God. Even if our bodies may not be perfect, because from imperfect humanity it is possible to produce an imperfect physical body, nevertheless we are never allowed to strip away the inherent dignity from humanity, at whatever stage we encounter it. **The only thing that can blemish or deform a soul is sin.** One, who has not yet been born, has not yet had the opportunity to actually sin by his/her own free will! He/she has only the corruption (Original sin) inherited from our first foreparents.

.When I was invited by a pro-life politician, along with two other Catholic physicians, to speak to the Federal Committee in Ottawa, looking into Organ Donation, one thing I found shocking was that another invited speaker, also a physician, when dealing with the issue of fetuses with physical defects, just matter-of-factly expressed the opinion that these fetuses be automatically aborted and used as a source of organs for donation (and these days, embryonic stem cells for research). Having delivered an anencephalic child, and having him baptized at birth, this physician's complete unawareness or dismissal of the dignity of humanity; the presence of a soul in the baby, notwithstanding the physical defect, was shocking to me. I know that I grieved the loss of my son, every bit as painfully as if he were physically normal. Even though I know and accept that he was too ill to live, I grieved his death, because HE , MY SON, EXISTED AS A HUMAN

BEING JUST AS REALLY AS MY DAUGHTERS AND I DO. In fact, this loss created a major spiritual crisis for me.

Knowing that we are born with the propensity to sin, God allows us, throughout our lives, many opportunities to repent and to amend our lives. We are told in Scripture that God has written His Law in our hearts and we know His Rules of Life. **Ezekiel 36: "I shall put My Spirit within you, says the Lord; you will obey My Laws and keep My Decrees;" and "I will put my Laws into their hearts and write them on their minds."[Heb 10:17]**.So, do other physicians believe that they have an eternal soul, as do all human beings from the first moment of conception until natural death, and do they care what happens to their souls after they die? This is for those who do believe or might want to think about it.

What motivated me to write and present this document, is that I think many physicians either don't know or no longer believe the above, admittedly very simplified version of our Salvation history. But even if they don't believe or remember, or have never connected their own personal and professional practices, with these basic rules, they all know they will die some day. What do they think happens then? Some people say they believe nothing at all exists after death. Do they believe in eternity and the four last things: death, judgment by God, and eternity in heaven or hell? Some think judgment and consequences is "an old wives tale." But only finding out when we get there, may be too late! To me, the reality of God's existence does not depend on whether or not we believe .

Many more don't believe hell exists either. However, it is a sobering thought that Our Lady of Fatima, now an approved Apparition in the Catholic Church,- a mission for repentance and conversion of humanity, at the beginning of the 20th century, did not hesitate, on the 13th July 1917, to show children aged 6, 7, and 10 at the time, a vision of hell, "where poor unrepentant sinners go," she said, so that we would believe in the existence of hell and do all we can to avoid ending up there. Jacinta, the youngest of the Fatima seers of our Lady, who died when she was ten during a stay in hospital in Lisbon, was disillusioned when she saw doctors whose only thought was of medicine and science exclusively, without any thought of God's part in healing. She once said, "Pity doctors; doctors do not know how to treat their patients with success because they have no love for God."(Msgr Joseph Cirrincione:*Blessed Jacinta Marto of Fatima.)*

The fact is that none of us have died and come back to tell the story. However, there are many, like myself, who have been in that corridor of death and been sent back. For most, that has been a life-changing experience. It is usually a change for the better-a conversion. There are many stories on websites from those who have had near-death experiences [NDEs];

they are mostly quite similar. [see International Association for Near Death Experiences IANDS and search www.NDEs].

Jesus Himself demonstrated the Truth about Life after death, first by raising Lazarus and others from death, then by His Own Resurrection. Furthermore, for the Truths He came to teach, the vast majority of His early disciples were martyred rather than waiver in their belief in Him. The story of the conversion of St Paul the Apostle stands out as a conversion experience and the transformation that ensued, from a foremost persecutor of the early Christians, to an ardent promoter and preacher of the Christian Faith after his encounter with the resurrected Christ. (Acts 9:1-30).But even before His Death and Resurrection we are given the profound eye witness report of His Transfiguration. In 2 Peter 1:16-19, we are told,"**We did not follow cleverly devised myths when we made known to you the power and coming of our Lord Jesus Christ, but we had been eyewitnesses of His majesty. For He received honour and glory from God the Father conveyed to Him by the Majestic Glory, saying, "this is My Son, My Beloved, with whom I am well pleased."** Mt 17:5 adds, "listen to Him." Among physicians, I'm afraid not many of us do even know these facts, let alone believe them or see any relevance in our lives.

Which one of us here does not already know how many doctors and their associated researchers, the scandal of Big Pharma falsified research results for the promotion of antidepressants,as well as selective publishing only of the research supportive of their drugs and the bribing of prominent psychiatrists also to promote especially the antidepressants etc., immoral research in third world or underprivileged societies such as India, are committing sins against human life, at the very beginnings of life, with ESCR, vaccinations from aborted embryos, *in vitro* fertilization, abortions, sex selection, contraceptives, morning after pills, genetic counseling for abortion, euthanasia, "mercy"killing, NHBD," brain death" when done by morally illicit organ procurement, transplant organs for money, body mutilation. Recently we also have the so-called human rights committees, trying to force doctors to park their morals (consciences) at the door,"to please patients and their demands when against the doctors' beliefs etc. Are these not "playing god?" By these acts, some of us are earning the "mark of Cain."(Gen 4:15). SOME but by no means all **"marks of Cain" Gen:4:15** are mentioned below.

1. Ethics

Since the abandonment of the Hippocratic Oath we now have this scenario where we have an endless gamut of so-called ethicists and ethics committees, coming up with their own "made to order" versions of what is right or ethical. How can they all be right? There is no standard course one takes to train to become an ethicist. It is the tower of Babel. (Gn 9:11) Again in Scripture, we are warned of these times (Mt 25:31-45) etc.

A few years ago I attended an ethics conference at which I heard the speaker proclaim, when she was asked at what stage she considered an embryo to be a fellow human being, that there were other equally important moral considerations! So, for instance, if a woman wants an abortion because she does not think she can afford to raise another child financially speaking, or the timing of the pregnancy is "inconvenient", these arguments should carry as much weight morally as the killing of the child? This, in spite of the fact that the fifth Commandment "Thou shalt not kill," stands with no qualifications whatsoever! [Ex 20:13].

Many think that if it is possible to do something it is automatically permissible to do it, especially since we have our own home made 'situational ethics committees' designed to vet and approve whatever we want in complete disregard of God's Commandments. In fact God is being disregarded and excluded almost everywhere in almost all walks of life, with fewer and fewer people praying or believing in Him or even considering His Commandments for a second, before acting. We would rather listen to our "false prophets."

At a workshop I gave about three years ago, along with 9 other members of The Association of Christian Therapists, we worked on the idea of an Oath that all God-fearing believers might be interested in hanging in our offices or workplaces, to replace the now largely abandoned Hippocratic Oath. I am aware that several other Oaths have been produced in the past but it seems none has really become very wide spread. As I group we believe that Life is still sacred and that we and all others of similar belief, must be seen to uphold the sacredness of life and honor God the Author of all life as stated in both the New and Old Testaments. The group were of varying backgrounds in religion; some Catholic, Christian, Jewish, Moslem, Sikh and no religion but people of good will. We came up with an Oath which can be seen and downloaded and printed for free at
It can be viewed at http://medial-oath.blogspot.com/
Some of you will recognize that the 8 statements on the Oath were the original work of the CHCW, used here with permission.

References.

1. **Humane Vitae**: Given at St. Peter's, Rome, on the 25th day of July, the feast of St. James the Apostle, in the year 1968, in the pontificate of Pope PAUL VI.
2. **Evangelium Vitae** : John –Paul PP II, 1995.03.25
3. **The Bioethics Mess** Dianne N. Irving, M.A., Ph.D. – in Crisis Magazine: Vol. 19, No. 5 May 2001).

There is a wealth of information available to flesh out the topics I have mentioned under "The marks of Cain" but I will briefly mention a few things on some. Those interested in these or related topics can research further information.

2. Religious and Human rights

Respect for human rights also includes protecting religious freedom, as a March 4 press release from the Organization for Security and Cooperation in Europe (OSCE) pointed out. The OSCE just held a meeting dedicated to the topic of intolerance and discrimination against Christians, the first OSCE meeting focusing specifically on the subject. Most if not all religions have felt discriminated against at some point.

"What came out clearly from this meeting is that intolerance and discrimination against Christians is manifested in various forms across the OSCE area, said Ambassador Janez Lenarcic, director of the OSCE Office for Democratic Institutions and Human Rights, which organized the meeting. Participants also highlighted inaccurate portrayals of Christian identity and values in the media and political discourse, leading to misunderstandings and prejudice, the press release explained. It's just over 60 years since, on Dec. 10, 1948, the U.N. General Assembly adopted the Universal Declaration of Human Rights. Then, as now, the need to protect basic liberties is an urgent task upon you and your families!

New Pro-Life, Christian Brand Offers Companies Method of Displaying Values Washington, DC (LifeNews.com) — Christian businesses wanting to display their faith and pro-life values now have a way to make that clear. The OVerus Christian Business emblem has received the okay for its official trademark registration from the United States Patent and Trademark Office. The emblem is a certification mark that represents Christian values and allows pro-life businesses to sort of wear their beliefs on their product. "This is a huge step forward for both the pro-life and Christian communities," Keith Miklas, founder and president of The OVerus Organization, tells LifeNews.com. He says the new emblem helps both pro-life businesses as well as customers and, once it has more of a national recognition and following, can help pro-life consumers discern which products and companies share their views. "Good Christian stewards can now easily select brands that respect their values, and brands have a way to distinguish their product or service to 208 million Christian shoppers," Miklas says. Full story at LifeNews.com

Human Rights in China —Population Control Continues To Claim Victims

By Father John Flynn, LC
ROME, JUNE 7, 2009 (**Zenit.org**) - China's human rights record was once more the focus of attention as June 4 marked the 20th anniversary of the bloody suppression of pro-democracy protests in Beijing's Tiananmen Square. The mainstream media focused on civil and political rights, but the

denial of the right of families to choose how many children they want continues to oppress many Chinese. On May 7, LifeNews.com published a report detailing the findings of an undercover investigation by Colin Mason in China. The fines for having an illegal child are now three to five times the family's income, LifeNews reported. Not surprisingly, when couples are faced with the prospect of such a fine, many consent to either abortion or sterilization. According to Mason, in Guangxi province babies born outside the government's limits are taken into custody by government officials, who hold the infants until the parents are able to pay the huge fines. On Feb. 15 the London-based Times newspaper reported that the government's severe restrictions are provoking widespread protests. According to the report, Chinese media and Internet commentators are breaking restrictions to report birth control abuses. Among the abuses, the Times mentioned that women who already have one child face regular pregnancy tests, as well as pressure to be sterilized. The means used to oblige women range from financial penalties to the threat of being sacked from their jobs.

Forced abortionOne case the Times mentioned was that of Zhang Linla, who committed the error of becoming pregnant when she had already given birth to a daughter. Just six days before the date she was due to give birth she was subjected to a forced abortion.The article mentioned other examples involving forced sterilizations and live babies being left to die.On Nov. 17 the Christian Post Web site reported on the case of Arzigul Tursun, a Muslim Uyghur woman who faced the threat of a forced abortion. At the time of the article she was more than six months pregnant and was being pressured by authorities to abort as she already had two children. On Oct. 5 the South China Morning Post newspaper published a lengthy article chronicling the coercive measures faced by couples not obeying the strict family planning laws. The article detailed the invasive nature of restrictions on families. Every married couple has to answer to the National Population and Family Planning Commission (NPFPC). Every village and every street in the cities are monitored by a family planning clinic controlled by the NPFPC.

According to the newspaper, there are officially 650,000 people employed to enforce the family planning laws. However, unofficial estimates say the real number is more than a million. The South China Morning Post gave the example of Jin Yani, who was subjected to a forced abortion due to her contravention of the strict limits. The abortion was carried out in such a brutal manner that she was in danger of death and subsequently spent 44 days in hospital. As a result of what happened, she will never be able to conceive again.

According to the article, authorities are able to act without scrutiny in the rural areas and they employ brutal methods, including the destruction of houses and forced sterilizations. The newspaper cited Mark Allison, East Asia researcher for Amnesty International, who said that forced abortions remain common.

Penalties

On May 22 the South China Morning Post reported that government authorities have renewed their determination to enforce strict family planning limits. Among the recent measures announced are the free distribution of contraceptives to migrant workers, and increased penalties for extra children. Revised family planning regulations released by the State Council announced that fines levied on migrant workers who violated the one-child policy would be assessed based on what they could earn in the place they are working, rather than the income levels of their hometowns. Setting the fine for breaking the family planning rule in the city where they are living in will result in higher penalties.

Incentives to follow official restrictions include extra holidays for those who wait until they are older to give birth, or who voluntarily undergo sterilization. Compliant couples will also receive preferential treatment from authorities when it comes to running their own businesses or receiving social relief. Such restrictions go against what the majority of Chinese women want, as even government officials admit. According to a Jan. 16 report by the BBC, Chinese family planning officials say their research shows that 70% of women want to have two or more babies. According to the BBC, the research was conducted in 2006, but has only been released now. Most women — 83% — want a son and a daughter, according to the survey.

<u>Missing girls</u> Apart from the abuses committed by authorities, another grave problem is a dangerous gap in the numbers of boys and girls being born. A combination of the traditional preference for having at least one male child, plus the restrictions on births, means that millions of baby girls have been aborted. According to an April 10 report by the Associated Press, the latest data reveals that China has 32 million more young men than young women. The estimate comes from a report published in the British Medical Journal. Moreover, the imbalance is expected to worsen in coming years. The study found that China has 119 male births for every 100 girls, compared with 107 to 100 for industrialized countries. The study found that the biggest boy-girl imbalance is in the 1- to 4-year-old group — meaning that China will have to face the effects of that when those children reach reproductive age in 15 to 20 years. Even though the government has banned the use of ultrasound tests to determine the sex of a fetus, they are still commonly done.

The consequences of a girl shortage are already being experienced, as the Sunday Times reported May 31. The London-based newspaper chronicled the increasing level of kidnappings of young girls. The girls are kidnapped to eventually be brides for men in regions where there is a severe shortage of girls being born.The article said that the public security ministry admits to between 2,000 and 3,000 children and young women being kidnapped each year, but local media put the figure as high as 20,000. A Web site established for parents to put up details of their missing children has information from more than 2,000 families. The hopes of resolving these kidnappings are, however, faint. After two years the site has had only resolved seven cases successfully.

Essential principles The anniversary of Tiananmen comes shortly after the United Nations commemorated the 60th anniversary of the Universal Declaration of Human Rights Archbishop Silvano Tomasi, the Holy See's permanent observer at the U.N. offices in Geneva, addressed the subject of human rights in a speech delivered Dec. 12."By speaking of the right to life, of respect for the family, of marriage as the union between a man and a woman, of freedom of religion and conscience, of the limits of the authority of the State before fundamental values and rights, nothing new or revolutionary is said," he commented. Human rights are not just entitlement to privileges, the Vatican representative pointed out. Unfortunately in China and other countries basic rights regarding the family are still not respected, a situation crying out to be rectified.

Medical workers deserve robust 'conscience clause' By James O'Neill
http://blogs.usatoday.com/oped/2009/04/medical-workers-deserve-robust-conscience-clause.html#more

Over three decades, Congress has passed laws (often collectively called the "conscience clause") that prohibit hospitals and other institutions that accept federal funds from forcing employees to act against their moral or religious convictions — such as providing sterilization or Plan B, or coercing them to perform or refer for abortions

Right to object

As a Department of Health and Human Services official, I discovered that many doctors didn't even know that they had the right to conscience protection. How could they be expected to defend such a right? In fact, a quasi-governmental certification organization, the American Board of Obstetrics and Gynecology, warned OB/GYNs in 2007 that "disqualification or diplomate revocation … may occur whenever" their practices conflict with the ethical code of the American College of Obstetricians and Gyne-

cologists, which proposed to add a requirement that "health care professionals have the duty to refer patients" to abortion providers, regardless of conscience objections.
James O'Neill was the principal associate deputy secretary of Health and Human Services in 2007-2008.

ALLIANCE FOR HUMAN RESEARCH PROTECTION
Promoting Openness, Full Disclosure, and Accountability
http://www.ahrp.org
FYI

The FDA is sliding rapidly down the slippery slope, abandoning widely accepted, international ethical research standards articulated in the internationally accepted Declaration of Helsinki—to facilitate commercial medical experiments.

An editorial by Dr. Michael Goodyear, of Dalhousie University (Canada), and a board member of The Alliance for Human Research Protection, provides an insightful explication of the moral significance of FDA's new rule lifting the requirement from clinical trials performed outside the US to conform to the Declaration of Helsinki when used to support applications for registration of products in the US. The Declaration is the primary source and arbiter of research ethics worldwide. It guides legislation and the ethical conduct and oversight of research, particularly in developing countries, which are the site of an increasing share of clinical research.

The move to accept the International Conference on Harmonization Good Clinical Practice (GCP) standards which are nothing more than procedural regulatory frameworks of the US, Japan, and Europe, is a backdoor tactic for reducing safeguards against exploitation of disadvantaged populations in underdeveloped countries. By withdrawing the Helsinki standards, FDA officials and industry are attempting to circumvent the Helsinki restrictions against use of placebos "where proven interventions" have been established. This restriction ensures that all human subjects are guaranteed current best therapeutic treatments against which the new experimental treatment would be tested. Industry much prefers to test new products against placebo—except in psychiatry where the placebo often as not proves as beneficial as the new drug, without the drug's hazardous side effects. [In the case of Eli Lilly's trial the placebo performed better than either its experimental antipsychotic (mGIu2/3) and its most profitable drug, Zyprexa) See:http://www.ahrp.org/cms/content/view/573/9/

High ranking FDA officials had waged a fierce but ultimately losing battle on behalf of industry to eliminate the restrictions on placebo when the Declaration underwent its 5th revision (2000) by the World Medical Association. However, as Dr. Goodyear points out, although the Declaration of Helsinki and the Nuremberg Code are not explicitly part of international or national law, their legal status is recognized. For example, both were cited by several US courts: TD v NYS Office of Mental Health (1995); Grimes / Higgins v Kennedy Krieger, Court of Appeals of Maryland (2001) http://www.courts.state.md.us/opinions/coa/2001/128a00.pdf ; and in the recent US Court of Appeals, which ruled that the Declaration (and other conventions) constituted a sufficient customary norm to be considered binding in the Pfizer trovafloxacin case in January 2009. The court reversed a dismissal by a lower court of a lawsuit by families of children who had died or were injured in a Nigerian meningitis trial.

The ethical principles articulated in the Declaration of Helsinki and the WMA's International Code of Ethics are morally binding on physicians: It is the duty of the physician to promote and safeguard the health of patients, including those who are involved in medical research. The physician's knowledge and conscience are dedicated to the fulfillment of this duty." [Principle 3] "It is the duty of physicians who participate in medical research to protect the life, health, dignity, integrity, right to self- determination, privacy, and confidentiality of personal information of research subjects." [Principle 11]The physician's moral obligation under the Declaration of Helsinki overrides local laws or regulations that may be governed by efficiency-based utilitarian standards. At a time of globalization, amidst growing concern about the political, social, and fiscal contexts in which biomedical research occurs, with its potential for power differentials and conflict of interest, the need for an international humanitarian standard of research ethics which (at least) holds physicians responsible for protecting the human subject, is even greater .Contact: Vera Hassner Sharavveracare@ahrp.org
212-595-8974

FAIR USE NOTICE: This may contain copyrighted (©) material the use of which has not always been specifically authorized by the copyright owner. Such material is made available for educational purposes, to advance understanding of human rights, democracy, scientific, moral, ethical, andsocial justice issues, etc. It is believed that this constitutes a 'fair use' of any such copyrighted material as provided for in Title 17 U.S.C. section 107 of the US Copyright Law. This material is distributed without profit.
http://www.bmj.com/cgi/content/short/338/apr21_1/b1559?rss=1
BMJ (British Medical Journal)April 21, 2009, 338:b1559 Editorial

Does the FDA have the authority to trump the Declaration of Helsinki? A new rule seems to be more about imperialism than harmonisation By Michael Goodyear, Trudo Lemmens, Godfrey Tangwa

The Food and Drug Administration (FDA) of the United States has ruled that clinical trials performed outside the US no longer have to conform to the Declaration of Helsinki if used to support applications for registration of products in the US. 1 Instead, the International Conference on Harmonisation Good Clinical Practice (GCP) has been designated as the new regulatory standard. This suggestion met considerable opposition from scientists, ethicists, and consumer groups before and during the consultations.[1] [2]

[3] The FDA's justifications included the arguments that it was merely harmonising its regulations with a global standard, and that legal instruments, such as the US Code of Federal Regulations, cannot embed external documents subject to change beyond the agency's control (dynamic referencing).[1] [4]

This justification failed to explain why GCP was any different in this respect, or why the declaration and the GCP were considered mutually exclusive. [2] Although such dynamic referencing can create legal problems,[5] [6] because legislatures cannot unreservedly commit to indefinite amendments, the declaration can, and should, be considered a minimum standard that reflects core ethical principles, operationalised through instruments such as the GCP and national regulatory policy. Static referencing of specific versions has not created substantial problems to date, and no reason is given about why this should be a problem now. The concerns remain unresolved, [7] but the question of what impact the change will make needs to be answered at both the instrumental (direct) level and the symbolic (indirect) level.

At first sight, the potential impact seems relatively small. Only a subset of clinical trials performed outside the US are affected, and supporters(mainly from industry) see the differences between the two documents as relatively minor. The real impact cannot be accurately ascertained at present, but it may be much greater than claimed because the US is the world's largest drug and medical device market. [7] In addition, increasing globalisation and movement of clinical trials "off shore" mean that a large proportion of such trials will be used in applications for marketing in the US.[8] [9] Some of the differences between the documents, such as those relating to the use of placebo controls in trials, are important and may have motivated the FDA to make this change. The fourth revision of the Declaration of Helsinki(1996) created difficulties for the FDA by restricting the use of placebos where proved interventions had become established. This had major implications for research in resource poor nations, where placebos were being used in such situations.[5] Despite heated debate,[10] the World Medical Association (WMA) has stood firm on the principle of not withhold in geffective interventions in its most recent (sixth) revision of 2008.[11] The FDA's decision therefore seems to reinforce its defence of placebo controlled trials.

Whatever the instrumental impact, in light of this history it is the symbolic aspects of the decision that should concern us most.[2] [8] T withdrawal of an unproblematic reference has far more significance than simply omitting it. We have grave misgivings about the future of international ethical norms, at least in the US. Despite assurances by the FDA, GCP is not an ethical code, but a procedural regulatory manual based on the regulatory frameworks of the US, Japan, and Europe. Thus, it is a description of existing procedures, not an aspirational document. It is not the procedural nuances that are at stake, but rather the moral reasoning that forms the basis of a culture of ethically responsible research. [5] [11] [12] The declaration, along with other international ethical guides, [5] remains a signpost for the collaborative development of international ethical principles and practice, the influence of which far exceeds national laws and regulations, and which was extended further in the2008 revision. The declaration is the primary source and arbiter of research ethics worldwide. It guides legislation and the ethical conduct and oversight of research, particularly in developing countries, which are the site of an increasing share of clinical research.

This symbolic move away from the declaration contrasts with its growing recognition elsewhere. Although not explicitly part of international or national law, the legal status of codes of ethical principles is recognised. The US Court of Appeals ruled that the declaration (and other conventions) constituted a sufficient customary norm to be considered binding in the Pfizer trovafloxacin case in January 2009.13 The court reversed a dismissal by a lower court of a lawsuit by families of children who had died or were injured in a Nigerian meningitis trial. The children had received this experimental antibiotic, and the court ruled that the declaration established a universal norm prohibiting non-consensual experimentation. Ata time of growing concern about the politics and increased globalisation of biomedical research, a more international view of research ethics is needed, rather than primacy of national policies that fall short of accepted principles. [9]

The FDA is at best acting as if its standards are distinct from globally accepted norms by pressuring the declaration to agree to its demands. At worst, it is creating an impression that it is more interested in facilitating research than respecting the rights of people who are the subjects of research. This has been variously depicted as entrenching different standards for different parts of the world (ethical pluralism),[5] [8] establishing the US's right to unique policies (exceptionalism), [2]and one country imposing standards on others (moral imperialism). [8] We must hope that the new administration in Washington will review the FDA's ill advised actions. [7]

The declaration and the WMA's International Code of Ethics contain the crucial statement that a doctor or investigator's conscience and ethical duty of care must transcend national laws. To be compliant with national laws that respect basic human rights and ethical norms is necessary, but is not in itself a sufficient standard How then can we best protect ethical principles in research? Historically, individual conscience, training, and ethical culture were considered sufficient. These have repeatedly fallen short of expectations, however, given the political, social, and fiscal contexts in which research occurs, with its potential for power differentials and conflict of interest. If organisations such as the FDA are unable or unwilling to foster an international culture of ethical research, it must fall to others, such as professional associations, to ensure that ethical reasoning is as central to research as it is to care,[10] and that ethical oversight has sufficient powers and resources to be effective. Although transgressions of ethical codes sometimes invite administrative and criminal sanctions, all professional associations have a responsibility to scrutinise the ethical competence, capacity, and practice of their members' research. Ultimately, ethically responsible research remains a collective responsibility. [5] Cite this as: BMJ 2009;338:b1559

Michael D E Goodyear, assistant professor of medicine1, Trudo Lemmens, associate professor of medicine and law2, Dominique Sprumont, professor of health law and deputy director3, Godfrey Tangwa, professor of philosophy4 1 Dalhousie University, Halifax, Nova Scotia, Canada B3H 2Y9, 2 University of Toronto, Toronto, Ontario, Canada M5S 2C5, 3 Institute of Health Law,University of Neuchâtel, 2000 Neuchâtel, Switzerland, 4 University of Yaoundé 1, PO Box 13597, Yaoundé, Cameroon mgoodyear@dal.ca Competing interests: None declared.
Provenance and peer review: Commissioned; not externally peer reviewed.

References

1. DHHS Food and Drug Administration. 21 CFR part 312. Human subject protection; foreign clinical studies not conducted under an investigational new drug application.
2. Final rule 28 April 2008, effective, October 27, 2008. , www.regulations.gov/fdmspublic/component/main?main=DocumentDetail&o=090000 64 80537f08.
3. Lurie P, Greco DB. US exceptionalism comes to research ethics.

Lancet2005;365:1117-9.[Cross Ref] [ISI][Medline]
4. Trials on trial: the Food and Drug Administration should rethink its rejection of the Declaration of Helsinki [editorial]. Nature2008;453:427-8.[Medline]
5. Normile D. Ethics. Clinical trials guidelines at odds with US policy.Science 2008;322:516.[Abstract/Free Full Text]
6. Goodyear MD, Krleza-Jeric K, Lemmens T. The Declaration of Helsinki. BMJ2007;335:624-5.[Free Full Text]
7. Sprumont D, Girardin S, Lemmens T. The Declaration of Helsinki and the law: an international and comparative analysis. In: Frewer A, Schmidt U,eds. History and theory of human experimentation: the Declaration of Helsinki and modern medical ethics. Stuttgart: Franz Steiner Verlag,2007:223-52.
8. Kimmelman J, Weijer C, Meslin EM. Helsinki discords: FDA, ethics, and international drug trials. Lancet 2009;373:13-4.[CrossRef][ISI][Medline]
9. Garrafa V, Lorenzo C. Moral imperialism and multi-centric clinical trials in peripheral countries. Cad Saude Publica 2008;24:2219-26.[ISI][Medline]
10. Glickman SW, McHutchison JG, Peterson ED, Cairns CB, Harrington RA,Califf RM, et al. Ethical and scientific implications of the globalization of clinical research. N Engl J Med 2009;360:816-23.[Free Full Text]
12. Lemmens T, Sprumont D, Nys H, Singh J, Glass KC. CIOMS' placebo rule and the promotion of negligent medical practice. Eur J Health Law2004;11:153-74.[CrossRef][Medline]
13. World Medical Association. Declaration of Helsinki. 2008. www.wma.net/e/policy/pdf/17c.pdf.
14. Goodyear MD, Eckenwiler LA, Ells C. Fresh thinking about the Declaration of Helsinki. BMJ 2008;337:a2128.[Free Full Text]
15. Abdullahi v Pfizer. US Court of Appeals 2d Cir. 2009 US App LEXIS 1768, 30 Jan 2009.

3. Embryonic Stem Cell Research, Abortion, IVF, Genetic counseling, Contraception, Morning after pills, Condoms.

Sometimes I contemplate how chaotic the universe would be if Our Lord granted the stars and moons and planets free will-if it would even exist at all any more, with each one choosing their own path and none sticking to the orbit or path designated to them. This is how human beings on earth are behaving. The result is chaotic killing of the vulnerable at every stage of life. Many nations have come to realize that the world is experiencing the graying of the planet, with a higher percentage of the living being now older and living longer, and fewer and fewer young people being born to replace them in the work place. We are facing our own destruction if not extinction, but many have still not realized this and are intensely focused on aborting the pre-born left, right and centre. A few governments are even trying to persuade families to have more children with not much success yet.

Today, 9th of March, 2009, as I begin this section, I hear on the news that President Obama is going to put into law the freedom to experiment on embryos, for the most part aborted embryos, our own little brothers and sisters whom we fail to or refuse to recognize and protect. Besides the shear horror of our sins, now worse than any holocaust, worse even than the sins of Sodom and Gomorra, I cannot help wondering about God's infinite Mercy to us, that He would still condescend to love us, and allow us to live, when He grieves the loss of so many of His precious Creations, destined to come to earth for His purposes, but obstructed or destroyed in the womb or before they even get there. Our hands are covered in blood, by acts we have legalized by and large throughout the world, with so few voices still raised in protest. The marks of Cain (Gn4:15) are upon many , if not most of us. Worse still, these actions are now so commonly done that we have lost a sense of sin and deadened our consciences, so we fail to see the effect sin is having on us.

http://www.ncbcenter.org/em/0908-1.aspx

ETHICS & MEDICS

AUGUST 2009 VOLUME 34, NUMBER 8

A Comprehensive Primer on Stem Cells *A stem cell is any cell that exists in a relatively immature state, and is able to divide to produce one cell that replaces itself and one that will go on to become a more specialized cell type. Because stem cells replace themselves every time they divide, they are considered self-renewing, or "immortal."

There are three broad classes of stem cells: embryonic, adult, and reprogrammed. Human embryonic stem cells are obtained by the destruction of human embryos that are between three and six days old. At this early stage, cells of the embryo are still very primitive and are pluripotent; i.e., they are able to produce all of the cell types found in the mature human body. In contrast, any stem cell that is found in a specific type of tissue (whether in an older embryo, a fetus, or a more mature individual) is considered an adult stem cell. Adult stem cells are thought to be more limited, making only the types of cells appropriate to the tissue in which they reside. Thus, they are seen as merely "multipotent." Finally, recent studies have shown that adult body, or "somatic," cells can be reprogrammed to a state very similar to a human embryonic stem cell. These induced pluripotent stem cells, or iPSCs,(1) are not identical to embryonic stem cells,(2) but they are functional equivalents; i.e., when transferred to early embryos, both cell types are able to produce all of the cells of the mature body.

How Useful Are They? Stem cells offer hope for treating medical conditions that are caused by a loss of cells, either due to injury or disease. To realize this hope, several important hurdles must be overcome. First, scientists must determine how to make stem cells mature into stable tissue that survives and functions normally. Second, stem cell derivatives must be safe for transplantation. Finally, scientists must find ways of effectively using stem cells to treat or cure medical conditions. Independent of the type of stem cell used for therapies, the pathology of many diseases is not sufficiently understood for stem cell treatments to be realistic; transplanted cells would simply fall victim to the same fatal influences that produced the disease initially. Thus, diabetes, Parkinson's disease, Alzheimer's, multiple sclerosis, and many other devastating conditions await a more thorough understanding of what causes cells to die before we can effectively treat patients with any type of stem cells.

In contrast, injuries such as those caused by heart attack or stroke present a more straightforward opportunity for stem cell therapies. In these cases, the approach to effective treatment (how to coax replacement cells into repairing damaged tissue) is likely to be similar, regardless of what kind of stem cell generates the replacement tissue. Therefore, to determine which stem cell type is likely to be the most useful, we need to ask, How do the three classes of stem cells compare in terms of the ability to produce stably differentiated cells that are safe for use in patients?

What Hope Do They Give? The serious safety issues raised by human embryonic stem cells have been discussed in detail.(3) Embryonic stem cells produce fatal tumors—indeed, such tumors are the gold-standard test for pluripotency. Embryonic stem cells can also convert to cancer cells.(4) In theory, both of these problems could be addressed by maturing embryonic stem cells into more stable cell types, yet this has proved to be very difficult, with even "differentiated" cells still producing tumors.(5) Despite more than a quarter century of research, the challenge of coaxing embryonic stem cells to form clinically safe cells has not been routinely overcome. Because cells derived from embryonic stem cells would be rejected by the immune system, human cloning has been proposed as a way to make patient-specific embryonic stem cells. However, cloned embryonic stem cells are known to be genetically abnormal, and this is not a simple problem to fix.(6) Thus, embryonic stem cells face serious and long-standing scientific hurdles before they can be safely used in patients.

In contrast to embryonic stem cells, adult stem cells have been used in clinics for decades. Stem cells from mature tissue (i.e., present at birth or later) do not cause tumors or convert to cancer.(7) Most (but not all(8)) adult stem cells divide more slowly than embryonic stem cells and have more restricted potency. However, some kinds of adult stem cells can differentiate into multiple cell types.(9) Importantly, because adult stem cells can be obtained from the patient, or "immune matched" from birth-related tissues like the umbilical cord and placenta, they will not be rejected.(10) These combined advantages have led to significant medical advances; adult stem cells have provided benefit for over seventy medical conditions in either animal or human studies,(11) and there are currently more than twenty-four hundred U.S.-funded clinical trials using adult stem cells.(12)

Reprogrammed iPS cells have some of the advantages of adult stem cells, and some of the disadvantages of embryonic stem cells. Like embryonic stem cells, iPS cells are pluripotent and therefore produce tumors. The early techniques used to generate iPS cells carried an increased risk of tumor formation, yet the iPS technique has been significantly improved. Current approaches have eliminated any added risk, and iPSCs are now no more likely to produce tumors or cause cancer than are embryonic stem cells. Just as for embryonic stem cells, it will undoubtedly be difficult to mature iPS cells into stable, functional cell types. However, initial studies suggest that this hurdle may not be as high for iPS cells as it is for embryonic stem cells.(13) Finally, iPS cells share with adult cells the advantage of being patient-specific. In the last year, scientists have produced a number of iPS cell lines from patients, to study specific diseases in the laboratory.(14) Thus, iPS cells are pluripotent (making them attractive for research), yet have the significant clinical advantage of being patient-specific.

The Ethics of Stem Cell Research Although production of human embryonic stem cells requires the destruction of nascent human life, some claim that the potential benefit to patients justifies this research. Yet, if embryos are human beings, arguing that it is permissible to destroy someone who is small and immature in the hope of benefiting someone of larger size or greater maturity is clearly an unethical line of reasoning. The critical question is whether human embryos are mere collections of human cells or developing human beings. And this question has been thoroughly addressed by the scientific evidence:(15) Embryos are developing human beings, not tumors or mere collections of human cells. They are small and immature, as all human beings once were, but they are human individuals. As Dr. Leon Kass, former chairman of the President's Council on Bioethics said, the moral issue does not disappear just because the embryos are very small or because they are no longer wanted for reproductive purposes: Because they are living human embryos, destroying them is not a morally neutral act. Just as no society can afford to be callous to the needs of suffering humanity, none can afford to be cavalier about how it treats nascent human life.(16)

Ethical objections to embryo-destructive research are based on religiously neutral reasoning that takes into consideration both the scientific evidence and current U.S. law regarding the protection of those who participate in experiments.(17) Protecting human research subjects is an important ethical consideration. The Nazi experiments on Jews, the Tuskegee syphilis experiments on black men, and the Japanese hypothermia experiments on prisoners of war were unethical and were not justified simply because they led to new and exciting discoveries that benefited patients. Science, like all human endeavors, must operate within an ethical framework. This is not a religious objection, it is just common sense.

Maureen L. Condic, Ph.D *Maureen Condic is an associate professor of neurobiology and anatomy at the University of Utah in Salt Lake City and a senior fellow at the Westchester Institute for Ethics and the Human Person in Thornwood, New York.*

1. K. Takahashi and S. Yamanaka, "Induction of Pluripotent Stem Cells from Mouse Embryonic and Adult Fibroblast Cultures by Defined Factors," Cell 126.4 (August 25, 2006): 663–676; and J. Yu et al., Induced Pluripotent Stem Cell Lines Derived from Human Somatic Cells," Science 318.5858 (December 21, 2007): 1917–1920.

http://www.ottawacitizen.com/opinion/flawed+quest+perfection/1868848/story.html **The flawed quest for perfection** Technology can eliminate many human imperfections, but we risk losing that messy quality that is the essence of our humanness By Margaret Somerville, Citizen Special August 7, 2009——The article starts with musings about home-knitted vs machine made sweaters, the latter being considered "better."

My musings about sweaters were prompted by thinking about the use of science in the search for human perfection. It is often said that nowhere are we at more ethical peril than when we undertake such quests. The Nazi horrors showed us the dangers of a political platform or public policy approach that uses science and technology to search for perceived biological "perfection" in ourselves, individually, and society as a whole. Today, we can seek the perfect baby through designing it using genetic and reproductive technologies — positive eugenics. The perfect copy of our self with cloning. The perfect war (risk free to us) with virtually controlled (disembodied) combat technologies. The perfect athlete with drug use or gene doping. The perfect body with cosmetic surgery.

Likewise, we can seek to eliminate those we see as imperfect — negative eugenics. We use new technology to carry out "embryo biopsies" (pre implantation genetic diagnosis) on in vitro fertilized embryos to identify and discard those who are "defective." We use prenatal screening to identify fetuses with genetic or other disabilities, such as Down's syndrome, and abort them. And, most recently, we have a do-it-yourself test that can be used at 10 weeks of gestation to see if the baby is male or female. If we are having a baby of the "wrong" sex, we can abort it and "try again."

And, in a context that is relevant to all of us because we will all face death, we can seek both to achieve the perfect death and to eliminate imperfect people through euthanasia and assisted-suicide.

I want to propose that these interventions in search of the perfect and to eliminate the imperfect threaten the essence of our humanness — our human spirit, that which makes us human and enables us to experience awe, wonder and the mystery of life, and through which we search for meaning. This latter search is of the essence of being human; we are meaning-seeking beings and, as far as we know, uniquely so.

Those who are religious define what constitutes the essence of our humanness as the soul — the sharing in a Divine spark. It is extremely difficult to define what constitutes that essence for those who reject religion, but many such people believe — or at least act as though — such an essence exists. For instance, anybody who agrees that humans are "special" as compared with other living beings and, therefore, deserve "special respect," is manifesting such a belief.

However, some secular humanists expressly reject such a belief. They regard "preferencing humans" (seeing humans as special as compared with other animals or even robots) as wrongful discrimination in the form of what they call speciesism. propose a very important question we need to ask in deciding what we may and should not do with our new technoscience, that is, what is ethical or unethical: Does any given use of this science, in the search for human perfection, damage or destroy the essence of our humanness? That leads to the question of whether at least some imperfections are elements of that essence and of immense value as such. Just like the hand-knitted sweater, are they part of what makes each of us unique originals?

I once wrote elsewhere that I wondered why seeing the original of a famous painting is not only different from, but much more exciting than, seeing an exact copy — at least, to me it is. (It turns out that some people prefer the copy. For instance, the Australian government built a replica of part of the Great Barrier Reef to reduce the number of tourists to the real reef in order to better protect it. Tourists from Japan preferred the replica to the real thing.)Or we can think about how antiques lose their value if they are refinished — when the many human hands that have touched the antique and the marks they have left have been erased, we consider that the antique is no longer authentic, that its priceless intangible essence is gone. In fact, we value such antiques less because in our later touching of them to alter them, they can no longer touch our imagination with the same profundity.

I believe that if we succeed in our search for human perfection — or, perhaps, even if we just engage in it — we will lose our authenticity, our human essence, our messy, old, much-touched soul. We will be like copies of masterpieces or like restored antiques: not originals, no longer unique, no longer the "real thing."Just as we changed our minds about which was the most valuable sweater, the perfect machine-made or the "imperfect" hand-knitted one, perhaps the same will happen with respect to our natural, untampered-with, imperfect human selves.

Margaret Somerville is director of the Centre for Medicine, Ethics and Law at McGill University, and author of The Ethical Imagination: Journeys of the Human Spirit.

© Copyright (c) The Ottawa Citizen

Embryonic Stem Cell Research Don't spread false hope about <u>embryonic</u> stem cell research .*National Post* Published: Tuesday, April 21, 2009 Re: Stem Cell Treatment To Tackle Blindness, April 20.

The hype generated around embryonic stem cells continues to grow out of control, judging by the National Post's front-page placement of the announcement of new British research study on age-related macular degeneration (AMD). Perhaps to counter the ethical darkness in using cells from aborted fetuses, the fawning publicity supporting embryonic stem cells has always far exceeded the reality.

In fact, there are exactly zero successful human treatments using embryonic cells. Despite the "huge step forward" headline, this news item is no exception. It merely announces that the multinational drug giant Pfizer has agreed to finance research trials which might lead to a human application "within seven years." Normally this would be covered in a one-paragraph item tucked back in the first section. Instead, the above-the-fold splash is sure to excite thousands of Canadian patients who might reasonably conclude that the Post would not make such a placement unless real patients had achieved real success. While one does not wish to dim anyone's hope, especially in this age of Obama, it must be tempered by reality. There are many, many hoops to go through, not least of which is the great difficulty in translating animal research on vision to a human therapy, especially one involving so delicate and precise a function as central vision. I have confidence that medical researchers will eventually develop ethically acceptable treatments for AMD and other tragic visual disorders. Until then, it is important that the media take seriously their role of balancing the value of truly newsworthy bioscience items against those that might lead to premature, even false, hope. Dr. Paul Ranalli, neuro-ophthalmologist, Toronto.

Washington, DC (LifeNews.com/CFAM) — Last week at a United States (US) House Foreign Affairs Committee hearing, Secretary of State Hillary Clinton stated that there was a new administration in place with different values, beliefs and global agenda. Nothing illustrated this rupture with previous U.S. policy more than her admission that the Obama administration interprets the term "reproductive health" to include abortion. In response to a question from Congressman Christopher Smith (R-NJ) on whether her definition of the phrases "reproductive health," "reproductive services," and "reproductive rights" includes abortion, Secretary Clinton stated that, "We [the current US administration] happen to think that family planning is an important part of women's health and reproductive health includes access to abortion that I believe should be safe, legal and rare." Clinton's linkage of family planning with abortion is not just a severe break with the previous administration; it is a clear violation of the Cairo Program for Action, which her husband's government helped to negotiate in 1994. The Cairo document explicitly states in two places that abortion should in no case "be promoted as a method of family planning." Full story at LifeNews.com

Obama to Sign Executive Order Monday Opening Public Funding of Embryonic Stem Cell Research which will open the door to direct taxpayer funds for embryonic stem cell research that encourages the destruction of human embryos is a slap in the face to Americans who believe in the dignity of all human life. Smith and the other pro-life Congressman observed that embryonic stem-cell research is not only unethical, but unnecessary, given the superior results achieved through adult stem cell research. "Human embryo-destroying stem cell research is not only unethical, unworkable and unreliable, it is now demonstrably unnecessary, Adult stem cells are truly remarkable. They work, they have no ethical baggage, and advances are made every day at a dizzying pace. But despite so much progress in the adult stem cell field, the Obama administration and the House and Senate Democratic leadership remain obsessed with killing human embryos for experimentation at taxpayer expense.If passed, the Freedom of Choice Act would enshrine abortion as a "fundamental right" that no government can "deny" or even "interfere with." This would immediately question the validity of all state and federal abortion regulations, including the partial-birth abortion ban, parental consent and notification laws, informed consent laws, and medical providers' legal right to refuse participation in abortion on moral grounds In light of this last threat, U.S. Catholic bishops have led the charge against the bill, citing their concern that Catholic hospitals across the United States would be forced to choose between disobeying the law and closing altogether. A grieving mother remembers differently,

"Like most Americans, January 20th, 2009 will be a day that is not soon forgotten in our household. However, it will be remembered differently for us. As I sat and listened to reporter after reporter gush about the championing of civil rights, I suffered the miscarriage of the little precious baby that we had only known for a matter of days was going to be a part of our family. Listening to the newscasts and mourning the loss of the life of our child gave me pause. Yes, Barack Obama is the first black President. But this election was by no means a triumph for inalienable rights. On the contrary, America successfully elected a black man who is more than willing to deny the most basic right to life itself of both unborn children (especially black children) and newly born children who survive an attempted abortion. Have Americans, liberals and conservatives alike, become so blind that they cannot see the forest for all of the trees?" Yes they have and not just Americans but much of the world.

President Obama's proposal to rescind a policy that protects the conscience rights of health care workers has now been formally published in the Federal Register, thus opening the 30-day period available for public comment on the proposal. Pro-life groups in the United States are urging concerned citizens to voice their concerns.The policy, one of the last acts of the Bush Administration, protects health care workers from being forced to perform and provide controversial services that conflict with their personal, moral and religious beliefs.

Pope Benedict XVI to the Participants in the Pontifical Academy for Life Symposium "Stem Cells: What Future for Therapy?"

Saturday, 16 September 2006

If there has been resistance — and if there still is — it was and is to those forms of research that provide for the planned suppression of human beings who already exist, even if they have not yet been born. Research, in such cases, irrespective of efficacious therapeutic results is not truly at the service of humanity. In fact, this research advances through the suppression of human lives that are equal in dignity to the lives of other human individuals and the lives of the researchers themselves.

History itself has condemned such a science in the past and will condemn it in the future, not only because it lacks the light of God but also because it lacks humanity.I would like to repeat here what I already wrote some time ago: Here there is a problem that we cannot get around; no one can dispose of human life. An insurmountable limit to our possibilities of doing and of experimenting must be established. The human being is not a disposable object, but every single individual represents God's presence in the world (cf. J. Ratzinger, God and the World, Ignatius Press, 2002).In the face of the actual suppression of the human being there can be no compromises or prevarications. One cannot think that a society can effectively combat crime when society itself legalizes crime in the area of conceived life. A good result can never justify intrinsically unlawful means. It is not only a matter of a healthy criterion for the use of limited financial resources, but also, and above all, of respect for the fundamental human rights in the area of scientific research itself.

I hope that God will grant your efforts — which are certainly sustained by God who acts in every person of good will and for the good of all — the joy of discovering the truth, wisdom in consideration and respect for every human being, and success in the search for effective remedies to human suffering. "We know already of Many successes/healings in the use of cord blood which now has its own banks, and adult human cells of many kinds (bone, skin etc) whereas not a single success in the use of ESCR (embryonic stem cell research) has yet produced any healing, not to mention the dangers which have not yet been overcome. And yet we have the following:President Obama, in his remarks on signing his <u>Executive Order on stem cells on March 9</u>, said that his decision "is about ensuring that scientific data is never distorted or concealed to serve a political agenda — and that we make scientific decisions based on facts, not ideology." He said that his Administration is committed to assuring that "our public policies [are based] on the soundest science; that we appoint scientific advisors based on their credentials and experience, not their politics or ideology; and that we are open and honest with the American people about the science behind our decisions."

The president spoke stirringly of the "urgent work of giving substance to hope and answering those many bedside prayers, seeking the day when words like 'terminal' and 'incurable' are finally retired from our vocabulary." Although earlier in this same address President Obama noted that "At this moment, the full promise of stem cell research remains unknown, and it should not be overstated ."Thus it is puzzling that the president's action revoked the 2007 Executive Order that had encouraged the National Institutes of Health [NIH] to support research to discover sources of pluripotent stem cells that do not involve destroying human embryos — that is, how to use ordinary adult cells to produce "induced pluripotent stem cells" (iPS).Because of this research, adult and cord-blood cells are now successfully being used to reverse serious illness, and to rebuild damaged organs. These striking developments in stem-cell research have been hailed by the journal *Science* as the greatest breakthrough of the past year. In addition, many scientists who specialize in this research have said that these iPS cells have *scientific* advantages over the stem cells derived from human embryos, making embryonic stem cells irrelevant to genuine medical progress. This would eliminate the serious ethical problem of destroying human embryos, and would overcome the "political" and "ideological" controversy that has surrounded this research.

We urge President Obama and his Administration's scientific advisors (Health and Human Services, NIH) to review his *Executive Order Removing Barriers to Responsible Scientific Research Involving Human Stem Cells*. As it stands, the new Executive Order forces all Americans to support research that destroys embryonic human life. Although the president laudably excludes human cloning (though no reason for this exclusion is given), his Order does not expressly favor the far more promising stem-cell research that does *not* involve the destruction of new human life, and which also has given far greater hope for finding cures. A review and refocusing of this Executive Order would help to achieve the president's goal to be "open and honest" about scientific facts, and his commitment to "make scientific decisions based on facts, not ideology". It would also help to answer the "bedside prayers" of countless Americans who cannot, in conscience, just

4. Prestigious Medical Journal Attacks Pope on Condoms

By Hilary WhiteMarch 31, 2009 (LifeSiteNews.com) - The Lancet, one of the medical world's most prestigious journals has accused Pope Benedict XVI of distorting scientific evidence to promote Catholic doctrine. Responding to the pope's comments that the use of condoms exacerbates the problem of HIV/AIDS in Africa, the Lancet called the pope's position, "outrageous and wildly inaccurate ."The editorial added, "By saying that condoms exacerbate the problem ... the pope has publicly distorted scientific evidence to promote Catholic doctrine. Whether the pope's error was due to ignorance or a deliberate attempt to manipulate science to support Catholic ideology is unclear."

"When any influential person ... makes a false scientific statement that could be devastating to the health of millions of people, they should retract or correct the public record. "However, supporters of the Pope have observed that the Lancet editorial contradicts the findings of research published in the magazine's own pages only two years ago. In the December 2007 edition of the journal, Dr. James D. Shelton of the US Agency for International Development, wrote that one of the "ten myths" about the fight against AIDS is that condoms are the answer. "Condoms alone," he wrote," "have limited impact in generalised epidemics."

A Harvard expert on AIDS prevention, Dr. Edward C. Green, who says he is an agnostic, recently told MercatorNet that the emphasis on condoms results not from the scientific evidence, but is driven by "ideology, stereotypes, and false assumptions." Dr. Green, the author of five books and over 250 peer-reviewed articles, said, "The Pope is actually correct. "He wrote in the journal First Things in 2008, that the determination by many in the international AIDS prevention community to push condoms results "in efforts that are at best ineffective and at worst harmful, while the AIDS epidemic continues to spread and exact a devastating toll in human lives."

Dr. Green's assertion coincides with the position of on-the-ground AIDS activists in Africa who have attempted to stem the flood of condoms into their countries, saying that it is sexual promiscuity that has increased AIDS in their countries. In 2008, Sam L. Ruteikara, the co-chair of Uganda's AIDS-prevention Committee wrote in the Washington Post that in the fight against AIDS, "profiteering has trumped prevention."

"AIDS is no longer simply a disease," he said, "it has become a multi-billion-dollar industry ... Meanwhile, effective HIV prevention methods, such as urging Africans to stick to one partner, don't qualify for lucrative universal-access status."

The Lancet's editorial is the latest in with what one British commentator called the "hysterical" reaction of much of the world's secular media to nearly everything the pope says, no matter how innocent. Kevin Myers, writing for the Belfast Telegraph, wrote, "Who would be Pope Benedict? The poor German has merely to say 'good morning', and the liberal tabloids are shrieking: 'Thousands dead in Sudan; famine across the world; ecological disaster everywhere - and Hitler Youth Pontiff thinks it's A GOOD MORNING!'" He continued, "What is it about sex which so diminishes rational thought?"

"Look. It's simple," Myers writes. "As part of an anti-Aids programme, condoms are unnecessary within a sexually continent people - Loreto nuns, say, or married couples who don't stray from the marital bed. "But condoms will not prevent the spread of Aids amongst a general population of sexually promiscuous individuals. Even if used conscientiously (which never happens in public health programmes) the best condoms in the world have a failure rate of around 5per cent."The result of this is the hard calculation, he says, that "actuarially", in every group of 20,000 people using condoms, at least 1,000 will fail. "In time, a very large number of the condom-using group will become infected by Aids. This is not a probability: it is an epidemiological certainty."

Dr. Laura Defends the Pope on the Condom FlapThe Pope, The Rabbi and Condoms by Dr.Laura Schlessinger

(Copyright 2009 by Take On The Day, LLC. Reprinted by permission.)April 3, 2009 (LifeSiteNews.com) - During his recent African trip, Pope Benedict XVI said that the distribution of condoms would not resolve the AIDS problem. The Pope has made it clear that abstinence is going to be the best way to fight AIDS. Google "Pope" and "condoms," and you'll never run out of reading material excoriating the man for his observation and opinion. Many health advocates have gone ballistic in their criticism of his comments. They feel it is one thing to promote abstinence as part of the Catholic religion, but that it is an entirely different thing to preach it to the world.

On a person-by-person basis, wearing a condom does, of course, offer some protection against contracting various venereal diseases and (of course) unwanted pregnancy. It is also true that condoms sometimes break, slip, or are put on incorrectly (taut to the very end). Everything has its limitations…except abstinence. I remember listening to a rabbi describing a situation that occurred to his kosher family. His 7 year old child was invited to a birthday party for a classmate at one of those fast-food hamburger establishments. When he came to pick up his child at the end of the party, one of the mothers - clearly annoyed - chastised him for the pain he caused his son. "All the children had hamburgers, chicken nuggets, french fries and dessert, and your little boy had to sit there and eat none of it. Imagine how terrible your son must have felt? How could you do this to him? Food is food. There is nothing sinful about food. What you are doing to him is just cruel." Just about at the end of her tirade, his son bounded up to him, gave him a huge hug around the waist, and said "I had a great time. This was a fun party."

The woman blanched and walked away. The rabbi followed her and gently told her the following: animals will eat whatever is around, even if it will make them unhealthy. Humans are to rise above animals and become masters of their urges. Imagine my son in a dorm room where harmful illicit drugs are being passed about. We already know that peer pressure and urges will not force him to relent and give in to the impulse. Learning at his early age to control impulse and desire is not a harmful trait - many times, it might be a life-saving one. Look at him. He enjoyed the company of your son and the rest of the children without giving up his values. He looks happy and satisfied. We really need to bring up our children to be masters of their instincts, not slaves to them, don't you think? The woman scowled, but listened to him.

Yes, in any one instance, a condom could protect, but in the overall scheme of humanity, why do so many people wish to push away the enormous protective power of moral values? When the Pope suggests that human beings are best off saving their sexual passion for the stability of a covenant of marriage, he is making a statement that the act of sexuality is elevated by the context, and ultimately protects both man and woman from a myriad of hurtful consequences from venereal diseases to unwanted pregnancies (complete with abortions, abandonment, single-parenthood, and homelessness to name a few). The naysayers all have one thing in common: they refuse to want, believe or accept that human beings can commit to a higher spiritual state of thought and behavior. The Pope believes in us more than that. I am not Catholic, so this is no knee-jerk defense of my spiritual leader. The truth is that he is simply correct and too many people don't want to hear it, because they want to live lives unfettered by rules. It is sad that they don't realize that this makes them a slave to animal impulse versus a master of human potential. see Dr. Laura's blog here: http://www.drlaurablog.com/

Listen to the Pope on Condom A response to: **Vatican Deplores Belgium's Criticism of Pontiff**

I am a Kenyan woman, a teacher, wife and mother. I fully support the Pope's message that condoms are not the solution to HIV/AIDS. With the promotion of condoms in my country, HIV/AIDS has only got worse. Let us listen to Pope Benedict. I wish I could shout, but I will not; but the truth

of the matter is that in my life I have not seen anybody more interested in the welfare of Africa than the Catholic Church. These other governments and organizations just talk for their own political correctness, hidden agenda and to defend all the myths they hold in their heads about Africa.Even before Pope Benedict said it, we knew the answer to HIV/AIDS and we agree with him, with clear minds.
Eme Oduor

Women for Faith & Family is an organization of Catholic women based in St. Louis, Missouri, representing about 50,000 Catholic women in the US and abroad.May 6, 2009**Statement of Women for Faith & Family on the National Institutes of Health Draft Guidelines for Human Stem Cell Research** (Implementing Executive Order 13505, March 9, 2009) Women for Faith & Family is deeply concerned about the draft guidelines for embryonic stem-cell research issued by the National Institutes of Health (NIH). Earlier legislation limited federally funded embryonic research only to frozen embryos, conceived through in-vitro fertilization (IVF), that the parents did not want. Though this destroyed new human life, the delay at least permitted the parents time to consider their actions. The proposed NIH guidelines go much further than previous legislation, and would open the door to even greater loss of life. The new guidelines would not restrict research to frozen "discarded" embryos, but would offer IVF parents the option to donate immediately their newly created embryos for destructive research, among other options for their "extra" (un-implanted) embryos. The NIH does not, in these proposed guidelines, allow the most extreme and radical ideas for human stem-cell research: namely, the creation of human embryos through somatic-cell nuclear transfer (i.e., cloning), and creating human-animal "hybrids". But this does not diminish the enormity of destroying countless human lives by government-supported researchers. Women for Faith & Family urges review of the draft guidelines, and the addition of an explicit preferential option for stem-cell research using mature (adult) stem cells, which has been far more productive of scientifically sound and medically useful results, and is ethically responsible since it does not destroy human lives.
Contact:
HelenHullHitchcock,Director;
Women forFaith&Family
POBox300411,St.Louis,Missouri,63130
Phone:314863-8385;Fax:314863-5858
E-mail:info@wf-f.org
Web site: http://www.wf-f.org1

5. Is Intravenous Fertilization Moral ?

http://www.stjoenews.net/news/2009/mar/08/beyond-octomom/
Beyond 'OctomombyErinWisdom Sunday, March 8, 2009 She's been splashed across newspapers, Web sites and television screens for more than a month now and, in the midst of this international media frenzy, has garnered a superhero-sounding name: Octomom. But Nadya Suleman has been made out to be more a villain than a hero, as a single, unemployed mother of six who chose to undergo in vitro fertilization and give birth to the eight children produced by it. In Missouri last week, Rep. Dr. Robert Schaaf, a Republican and a St. Joseph physician, proposed state legislation that would limit the number of embryos implanted during IVF, thereby preventing women here from following in Ms. Suleman's footsteps. This suggested measure is just one example of how, as much in the spotlight as she is, Ms. Suleman really is at the heart of a much bigger issue — one concerning the ethical issues raised by the industry that enabled a situation like hers in the first place.

"These IVF physicians need to have the living daylights regulated out of them," says Dr. Sarah Breir, associate director of the University of Missouri School of Medicine's Center for Health Ethics. "We've let technology get beyond the regulations to control it."Although the American Society of Reproductive Medicine and the Society for Assisted Reproductive Technology have created guidelines for the number of embryos implanted during IVF — ranging from no more than two for women 35 and younger to no more than five for women 40 and older — physicians have the freedom to deviate from these. Ms. Suleman, 33, had six embryos implanted, and two split into twins.

Implanting such a large number of embryos goes against a doctor's duty to "do no harm," Dr. Breir says."It's incompatible with a safe and reasonable expectation of pregnancy. A mom and her healthcare team have ethical duties to try to maintain a gestational period of 40 weeks," she adds, which just isn't possible for a woman pregnant with multiples.Another issue highlighted by Ms. Suleman's case is the fact that today's IVF procedures often result in embryos that are destroyed. Ms. Suleman's octuplets, it has been reported, were frozen embryos left over from previous IVF treatments that would have been destroyed had she not had them implanted. Later, when multiple fetuses were detected, she refused to undergo selective reduction.

"Selective reduction is just another way of saying abortion," Dr. Brier says, "and I think we need to question whether women who are implanted with multiple embryos are fully informed that they might face that decision. Most wouldn't want to look at an ultrasound and say, 'Kill this one and this one and this one.'"Despite these ethical concerns, Dr. Brier isn't against IVF; she simply thinks it should be regulated to the point that so many embryos aren't being created and then either destroyed or implanted in numbers that aren't safe for the mother and babies. But to some, even regulations such as these wouldn't be enough to make IVF ethical.

"The attitude that couples take on when they pursue IVF thwarts God's plan for each child to be brought into this world through a sexual act of total and committed love between married parents," says Adrienne Doring, director of the Catholic Diocese of Kansas City-St. Joseph's Respect Life office. "Every child should have the dignity of being created through an act that its mother, father and Creator participate in — rather than taking the act from the bedroom to the laboratory and placing conception in the hands of a scientist."

This issue is just one — in addition to those surrounding the fate of "extra" embryos — that the Catholic Church has with IVF. But this doesn't mean the Church doesn't sympathize with couples struggling with infertility, Ms. Doring adds. Rather, it strives to offer solutions through Natural Procreative (NaPro) Technology, which works to resolve the issues at the root of infertility. This might include using surgery to correct problems or supporting a pregnancy with progesterone in order to help a married couple conceive and carry a child to term, Ms. Doring says, noting that these methods have been shown to have a higher success rate than IVF.

Pinpointing the cause of a fertility problem and then treating it can take months or even years — a wait that, of course, can be difficult for a couple who are ready for a baby now. But the wait required to treat fertility problems naturally is worth it, says Marla Daugherty of St. Joseph, in that this method addresses root issues rather than bypassing them. "It goes deeper than helping a couple have a baby," says Ms. Daugherty, who works as a practitioner with FertilityCare Center of Kansas City, which uses NaPro Technology.Through monthly classes offered at (but not affiliated with) Heartland Regional Medical Center, Ms. Daugherty helps women learn to chart their cycles — sometimes as a means to naturally avoid or achieve pregnancy and other times as a way to collect data doctors can use to identify hormonal problems that could be causing infertility."Women suffer from this," Ms. Daugherty says. "When we look at them, we care not just about helping them achieve pregnancy but also about treating them for what they're suffering."Lifestyles reporter Erin Wisdom can be reached at ewisdom@npgco.com.

CMAJ article on Prenatal DNA test - "Is this a new eugenics?" asks Somerville

All editorial matter in CMAJ represents the opinions of the authors and not necessarily those of the Canadian Medical Association.

Prenatal DNA test raises both hopes and worries
Roger Collier ,CMAJ.

Twenty-one weeks into her pregnancy, Barbara Farlow discovered that her daughter Annie would be born with the genetic disorder trisomy 13, a chromosomal abnormality — and a label — that would determine her future medical care.

In August 2005, Annie, not yet 3 months old, suffered a respiratory attack and was admitted to hospital. She died within 24 hours. The official cause was "complications of trisomy 13," but Farlow and her husband still don't know the details, despite years of inquiry. They do know, however, that someone issued a do-not-resuscitate order without their consent.

"I feel that the genetic testing ultimately determined her fate," says Farlow, who lives in Mississauga, Ontario. "She was treated as a syndrome. She wasn't treated as a child."

A new prenatal genetic diagnostic test may soon cause a substantial increase in the number of fetuses affixed with "syndrome" labels. The noninvasive test, called chromosomal microarray analysis, allows doctors to detect submicroscopic genetic abnormalities that no other test can find. Advocates of the technology say it is safer, faster and more accurate than invasive diagnostic procedures like amniocentesis. Despite the test's benefits, however, some worry that it will result in a flood of prenatal genetic information of uncertain significance and will lead only to confusion and undue anxiety for expectant parents. Others question whether scientists should even be in the business of cleaning up the gene pool and have evoked the dreaded "E" word: eugenics.

Researchers have been able to diagnose certain genetic conditions, like Down syndrome, in fetuses since the 1960s. This has traditionally been done through karyotyping, which involves extracting cells from amniotic fluid, culturing and staining them in a lab, and examining them under a microscope. In microarray testing, fetal DNA is obtained from a pregnant woman's blood. This eliminates the need to perform amniocentesis, a test that slightly increases the risk of miscarriage. The fetal DNA is compared to control DNA stored on a "gene chip." It detects chromosomal anomalies 100 times smaller than those revealed by traditional tests.

"I think there's going to be a major change in the way prenatal diagnosis is done," says Dr. Arthur Beaudet, chairman of the Department of Molecular and Human Genetics at Baylor College of Medicine in Houston, Texas. "It's cost-effective if couples are going to terminate. For children born with severe disabilities, their lifelong care is very expensive." Baylor is one of the few institutions openly promoting microarray testing (others include Signature Genomic Laboratories in Spokane, Washington, and Emory University in Atlanta, Georgia). No Canadian lab yet offers the test, though doctors can order it from the United States. Beaudet says the biggest barriers to widespread adoption of the test are its cost (US$1600) and the reluctance of US insurance companies to cover it. "My goal is to get the cost of a new test down to the cost of current tests, and to encourage insurance providers to offer to pay for the new test or the old test, but not both. I hope that's where we are a year from now."

Microarray testing has already been used extensively as a diagnostic tool in pediatrics. When used to identify the genetic roots of mental retardation in children, for instance, it has proven twice as effective as conventional techniques. Researchers say it may be even more useful for prenatal diagnosis, detecting up to 200 genetic abnormalities, while returning ambiguous results in only 1% of cases. Proponents of the test also point out that it can be performed earlier than amniocentesis and that it provides the maximum amount of information about a fetus, allowing a prospective parent to either terminate the pregnancy or prepare for a child with disabilities. "For detecting fetal abnormalities, there is no doubt that microarray is a very useful technique," says Dr. Doug Wilson, who heads the Department of Obstetrics and Gynecology at the University of Calgary, in Calgary, Alberta.

Some genetic researchers believe it is premature to promote widespread use of microarray testing. The chromosomal imbalances that the test detects are so subtle that interpreting their significance is difficult. Doctors cannot tell their patients definitively if some detected anomalies are benign or pathogenic. They will not necessarily know the impact of an abnormality, or its severity, if one exists. Will fetuses with relatively minor genetic defects — an increased risk for cancer, say, or a predisposition toward obesity — be regularly aborted? "This detects way more than has ever been detected before, and has moved from research to clinical practice very quickly," says Dr. Jan Friedman, professor of medical genetics at the University of British Columbia in Vancouver, British Columbia.

Friedman recognizes the strengths of microarray testing but warns that nobody's DNA, when you dig deep enough, is perfect. Subtle genetic variations are normal and often harmless. Friedman recommends that the technology only be used, at least for now, in clinical trials or for pregnancies in which fetuses are at high risk of having chromosomal abnormalities. Because couples can terminate a pregnancy early in the term for any reason, Friedman says, doctors will be dealing with that issue more if microarray testing becomes popular, and they should not ignore the effects of dropping mountains of genetic data onto people's laps. "It behooves us to give this some thought before we reach that point."

If the test does become commonplace — and it soon will, according to some geneticists — providing good genetic counselling to expectant parents will be crucial. Understanding complex and sometimes ambiguous genetic information is no easy task. Many people don't even know the difference between risk and diagnosis. The primary challenge that microarray testing will present, however, may not be understanding the data but just getting through it. "For me, the difference is the volume of the information you are getting," says Chris Trevors, board secretary of the Canadian Association of Genetic Counsellors. "People look for health care providers to guide them on how to interpret this info, and if we can't, I don't think we should be offering it."

Then there are the ethical concerns. Medical ethicists and disability rights advocates question the motivations behind promoting microarray testing. There are no treatments for many of the genetic disorders the test will uncover. That leaves termination as the only option for parents who don't want disabled children. Disability support groups cite the effect of prenatal screening for Down syndrome as the most ominous example — the number of children born with the condition dropped by almost 90% when screening for it became widespread. Do we want a society, some ask, in which disabled people will eventually be found only in history books?

"There's a biological imperative for diversity. If we eliminate things like Down syndrome, what else is next?" asks Krista Flint, executive director of the Canadian Down Syndrome Society. Advocates for the test say expectant parents can never be too informed and that more knowledge empowers people to make better choices. But detractors warn that it's folly to ignore the collective impact of individual choices and that nothing good has ever come from the scientific pursuit of human perfection.

"Are we on a search-and-destroy mission for babies that don't measure up?" asks ethicist Margaret Somerville, Samuel Gale Professor of Law at McGill University in Montréal, Quebec. Some claim doctors favour microarray testing because it provides better protection against wrongful-birth lawsuits, which ethicists say is an inappropriate benchmark for setting standards of care. Evelyne Schuster, medical ethicist at the University of Pennsylvania, in Philadelphia, Pennsylvania, has said that normality cannot be established at the molecular level. Adrienne Asch, director of the Center for Ethics at Yeshiva University, in New York, has expressed concern that a time will come when all parents genetically audition their fetuses to determine if they are worthy of life.

6. Vaccination: Grateful thanks for the tireless work of Debbie Vinnedge and associates, the faithful watchdogs who update and maintain the Website at "Children of God for Life."

US AND CANADA - ABORTED FETAL CELL LINE PRODUCTS AND ETHICAL ALTERNATIVES
Updated:

Disease	Product Name	Manufacturer	Fetal Cell Line	Ethical Version	Manufacturer	Cell Line
Chickenpox	Varivax, Varilrix	Merck, GSK	WI-38, MRC-5	None	N/A	N/A
Hepatitis A	Vaqta, Havrix Avaxim, Epaxal	Merck, GSK Sanofi, Berna	MRC-5 MRC-5	Aimmungen Not available in US	Kaketsuken (Japan & Europe)	Vero (monkey)
Hepatitis A & B	Twinrix	GSK	MRC-5	Engerix Hep-B Only	GSK	Yeast
Hepatitis A & Typhoid	Vivaxim	Sanofi	MRC-5	Recombivax Hep-B Only	Merck	Yeast
Measles/Mumps/Rubella	MMR, Priorix	Merck, GSK	RA273, WI-38	None	N/A	N/A
Measles-Rubella	MR Vax Eolarix	Merck GSK.	RA273, WI-38 RA273, MRC-5	Attenuvax (Measles Only)	Merck	Chick embryo
Mumps-Rubella	Biavax II	Merck	RA273, WI-38	Mumpsvax (Mumps Only)	Merck	Chick embryo
Rubella	Meruvax II	Merck.	RA273, WI-38	Takahashi Not available in US	Kitasato Institute (Japan & Europe)	Rabbit
MMR + Chickenpox	ProQuad/MMR-V	Merck.	RA273, WI-38, MRC-5	None	N/A	N/A
Polio	Poliovax, DT Polio Adsorb.	Sanofi Pasteur	MRC-5	IPOL	Sanofi Pasteur	Vero (monkey)

Disease	Product Name	Manufacturer	Fetal Cell Line	Ethical Version	Manufacturer	Cell Line
Polio Combination (DTaP + polio+ HiB)	Pentacel Quadracel	Sanofi Pasteur	MRC-5	Pediacel; Pediarix + HiB Infanrix Hexa + HiB IPOL + any DTaP + HiB	Sanofi, GSK	Vero (monkey)
Rabies	Imovax	Sanofi Pasteur	MRC-5	RabAvert	Chiron	Chick embryo
Rheumatoid Arthritis	Enbrel	Amgen	WI-26 VA4	Humira	Abbott Labs CH	Hamster Ovary
Sepsis	Xigris	Eli Lilly	HEK-293	Ask your doctor	N/A	N/A
Shingles	Zostavax	Merck.	WI-38, MRC-5	None	N/A	N/A
New: Smallpox	Acambis 1000	Acambis	MRC-5	ACAM2000, MVA3000	Acambis/Baxter	Vero, Chick Embryo
In Development Ebola	TBA	Crucell/NIH	PER C6	None	N/A	N/A
In Development Flu, Avian Flu, Swine Flu	TBA	Vaxin, Sanofi	PER C6	All current flu vaccines New Flu, Swine & Avian Flu in development	Medimmune, Novartis, CSL Ltd, ID Biomed, Sanofi, GSK, Chiron Novavax, Protein Sci., Novartis, MedImmune, Baxter	Chick embryo Insect, Caterpillar, MDCK, MDCK, Vero
In Development: HIV	MRKAd5 HIV-1	Merck	PER C6	None	N/A	N/A

— 41 —

Note: Immune-Globulin shots will provide temporary immunity (4-6 months) for Hepatitis-A and Rubella (3 months)
Physician Order: Merck: 800-422-9675 GSK: 866-475-8222 Sanofi Pasteur: 800-822-2463 Chiron:(800 244-7668 (PST)
NOTE: ANY VACCINE NOT LISTED ABOVE DOES NOT USE ABORTED FETAL CELL LINES.

Use of Human Cell Lines in Pharmaceuticals – Canada see below page 35.

Various commercially available pharmaceutical products are derived from or cultivated on fetal cells lines that were obtained from abortions. Patients may have a biological, ethical or religious objection to products that come from human sources. The chart below allows us to provide information to patients to make informed decisions. It also makes known the fact the alternatives are available in other countries and should be available in Canada.

NOTE: -All flu vaccines use non-human cell lines
-Immune-Globulin shots will provide temporary immunity (3-5 months) for Hepatitis-A and Rubella

Disease	Drug Name	Manufacturer	Cell Line (Fetal)	Alternative (Drug/ Manufacturer /Source)
Chickenpox	Varilrix ®	GSK	MRC-5	**None**
	Varivax®	Merck & Co	WI-38, MRC-5	**Available**
Hepatitis A	Epaxal®	Berna Biotech	MRC-5	Aimmungen®
	Havrix ®	GSK	MRC-5	Kaketsuken
	Vaqta ®	Merck & Co	MRC-5	Vero (monkey)
	Avaxim ®	Sanofi Pasteur	MRC-5	**Available in**
	Avaxim Pediatric ®	Sanofi Pasteur	MRC-5	**Japan and Europe**
Hepatitis A and Typhoid Fever	Vivaxim ®	Sanofi Pasteur	MRC-5	**As above for Hep A component**
Hepatitis A & B	Twinrix ® (Hep A Component)	GSK	MRC-5	**As above for Hep A component, Hep B is derived from yeast**

Disease	Drug Name	Manufacturer	Cell Line (Fetal)	Alternative (Drug/ Manufacturer /Source)
Measles, , Mumps Rubella	Priorix ® MMR II ®	GSK Merck & Co	MRC-5 RA27/3, WI-38	Attenuvax® (Measles) Merck Chick embryo **Availabe in US** Mumpsvax ® (Mumps) Merck Chick embryo **Available in US** Takahashi (Rubella) Kitasato Institute Rabbit **Available in Japan and Europe**
MMR + Chickenpox	ProQuad ®	Merck & Co.	RA27/3, WI-38, MRC-5	**None Available**
Polio	Inactived Poliomyelitis Vaccine – IPV ® Pentacel ® Quadracel ® Td Polio Adsorbed ®	Sanofi Pasteur	MRC-5	Infanrix-IPV, Infanrix Hexa & IPV/Hib® GSK (Europe) Vero Cells **Pediacel to be offered in Alberta March 2007**
Rabies	Imovax ®	Sanofi Pasteur	MRC-5	Rabavert® Chiron Chick Embryo **Available in Canada**
Rheumatoid Arthiritis	Enbrel ®	Immunex (Amgen)	WI-26 VA4	**None Available**
Sepsis	Xigris ®	Eli Lilly	HEK-293	**None Available**

Reference:
1. Varilirix Product Monograph. GlaxoSmithKline Inc. http://www.gsk.ca/en/products/vaccines/varilrix_pm.pdf. Accessed March 14, 2006.
2. Varivax. Product Monograph. Merck. http://www.merck.com/product/usa/pi_circulars/v/varivax/varivax_pi.pdf. Accessed March 14, 2006.
3. An Advisory Committee Statement (ACS) National Advisory Committee on Immunization (NACI). Supplementary Statement On Hepatitis A Vaccine (Acs-4). http://www.phac-aspc.gc.ca/publicat/ccdr-rmtc/00vol26/26sup/acs4.html. Accessed March 14, 2006.
4. Vaqta Product Monograph. Merck. http://www.merck.com/product/usa/pi_circulars/v/vaqta/vaqta_pi.pdf Accessed March 14, 2006.
5. Havrix. Product Monograph. GlaxoSmithKline Inc. http://www.gsk.ca/en/products/vaccines/havrix_pm.pdf. Accessed March 14, 2006.
6. Priorix Product Monograph. GlaxoSmithKline Inc. http://www.gsk.ca/en/products/vaccines/priorix_pm.pdf. Accessed March 14, 2006.
7. MMR II Product Monograph. Merck. http://www.merckfrosst.ca/e/products/monographs/M-M-R_II-756-a_3_02-E.pdf. Accessed March 14, 2006.
8. ProQuad Product Monograph. Merck. http://www.merck.com/product/usa/pi_circulars/p/proquad/proquad_pi.pdf . Accessed March 14, 2006.
9. IPV Product Monograph. http://www.vaccineshoppecanada.com/secure/pdfs/ca/ipv_E.pdf . Accessed March 14, 2006.
10. Imovax Product Monograph. http://198.73.159.214/statics/vaccines/english/IMOVAX_E.pdf. Accessed March 14, 2006.
11. Enbrel. United States Patent. http://patft.uspto.gov/netacgi/nph-Parser?Sect1=PTO1&Sect2=HITOFF&d=PALL&p=1&u=/netahtml/srchnum.htm&r=1&f=G&l=50&s1=5,712,155.WKU.&OS=PN/5,712,155&RS=PN/5,712,155. Accessed March 14, 2006.
12. Vaccines And Related Biological Products Advisory Committee. United States Of America Food And Drug Administration Center For Biologics Evaluation And Research. http://www.fda.gov/ohrms/ dockets/ac/01/transcripts/3750t1.rtf . Accessed March 14, 2006.
13. Jacobs JP, et al. Characteristics of a human diploid cell designated MRC-5. *Nature*. 1970;227(5254):168-70.
14. Plotkin SA, Cornfield D, Ingalls TH. Studies of Immunization with living rubella virus: Trials in children with a strain cultured from an aborted fetus. *Am J Dis Child.* 1965;110: 381-389.
15. Plotkin S, et. al. Attenuation of RA27/3 Rubella Virus in WI-38 Human Diploid Cells. *Am J Dis Child.* 1969;118:178-185.
16. Weibel RE, et al. Clinical and laboratory studies of combined live measles, mumps, and rubella vaccines using the RA 27/3 rubella virus. *Proc Soc Exp Biol Med*. 1980:165(2):323-326.

17. Hayflick L, et al. The serial cultivation of human diploid cell strains. *Exp Cell Res.* 1961;25:585-621.

The Merck Boycott

For over 30 years Merck has been using aborted fetal cell lines in the production of vaccines, despite the fact that there are ethical alternatives that could be used. Further, when pressed to cease this immoral, unnecessary practice, Merck assured the American public that "No further fetal tissue would be needed now or in the future to produce vaccines." They have broken that promise by contracting with Dutch Biopharmaceutical company, Crucell NV, for use of their new aborted fetal cell line, PER C6 - taken from the retinal tissue of an 18-week gestation baby, which will be used in their new HIV vaccine. Not only do they refuse to listen to the voice of over half a million Americans who have written to protest, they continue to exploit our unborn and profit from the destruction of innocent human life. Pro-life America has had enough! If you agree, please join our fight.

Following is a list of Merck's major drug products -
and their competitor's.
We strongly recommend you check with your doctor to be sure the alternative products are appropriate for your personal medical condition. If so, use them - and let your doctor know why! And let Merck know why too! Write to:
Richard Clark, Residing Chairman -
Merck & Co.
770 Sumneytown Pike
P.O. Box 4
Westpoint, PA 19486

NOTE: We realize there are companies listed below that may or may not be any better than Merck when it comes to unethical practices. We do hope though that if you have to choose one evil against another, you won't choose Merck - until they agree to live up to the high standard of ethics they profess to have.

MERCK PRODUCT	COMPETITOR	PRODUCT NAME	CONDITION
AGGRASTAT® (tirofiban HCl)	Schering-Plough	Integrelin	Used to decrease chances of clots after certain cardiac events.
CANCIDAS® (caspofungin acetate)	None	None	Aspergillus fungal infection
COMVAX® Haemophilus B Conjugate and and Hepatitis-B (Recombinant) Vaccine]	Wyeth, Aventis Glaxo SmithKline	Separate Doses: Hib: HbOC, ActHib Hepatitis B: Engerix	Haemophilus B Hepatitis B
COSOPT® (ophthalmic solution)	Allergan Alcon	Betagan, Aphagan Timolol Betimol	Glaucoma
COZAAR® (losartan potassium)	Novartis Unimed Sanofi-Synthelabo Boehringer Ingelheim Sankyo	Diovan Tevetan Avapro Micardis Benicar	Blood Pressure Prevention of nepropathy in certain diabetics Prevention of stroke
CRIXIVAN® (indinavir sulfate)	Agouron Abbott Roche	Viracept Norvir Fortovase (Saquinavir)	AIDS
FOSAMAX® (alendronate sodium tablets)	Proctor & Gamble Roche/GSK	Actonel Boniva	Osteoporosis
HYZAAR® (losartan potassium and hydrochlorothiazide)	Novartis Bristol Myer Squibb Sankyo Boehringer Ingelheim Unimed	Diovan HCT Avalide Benicar HCT Miacardia HCT Teveten HCT	High Blood Pressure
MAXALT® (rizatriptan benzoate) and Maxalt MLT®	AstraZaneca Elan Pfizer	Zomig Frova Relpax	Migraine Headaches
PedvaxHIB® Haemophilus B Conjugate Vaccine (PRP-OMP)	Aventis Pasteur	ActHIB	H-Type Flu

MERCK PRODUCT	COMPETITOR	PRODUCT NAME	CONDITION
PEPCID® COMPLETE	Apotex Eli Lilly Others	Ranitidine Axid Generics: Famotidine, Ranitidine, Nizatidine, Cimetidine	Ulcers, GERD, erosive esophagitis, heartburn
PNEUMOVAX® 23, Pulmovax (Pneumococcal Vaccine)	Wyeth	Prevnar Pnu-Immune 23	Pneumonia
PROPECIA® (finasteride)	None	None	
PROSCAR®	Boehringer Ingelheim Glaxo SmithKline Abbott Pfizer Pfizer	Flomax Avodart Hytrin Cardura Minipress	Symptoms of BPH
RECOMBIVAX HB® [Hepatitis B Vaccine (Recombinant)]	Glaxo SmithKline	Engerix	Hepatitis-B
SINGULAIR® (montelukast sodium)	AstraZeneca Abbott	Accolate Zyflo	Allergies, Asthma
VIOXX ®	Pfizer Pharmacia Boehringer	Celebrex Bextra Mobic	Certain types of arthritis, Anti-inflammatory
Zocor®	Pfizer Bristol Meyers- Squibb AstraZeneca Novartis Generic Kos Pharma	Lipitor Pravachol Crestor Lescol XL lovastatin Altoprev	Used to lower cholesterol and lipids

8. Abortion :
Yes, animals feel pain, but preborn children feel pain too during lethal abortion procedures

For Immediate Release September 28, 2009

OTTAWA – Just prior to MP Maurice Vellacott tabling petitions today, Liberal MP Marlene Jennings tabled a petition calling on the government to adopt effective animal welfare legislation because "It is well known that there is scientific consensus and public acknowledgement that animals feel pain and can experience suffering."

Vellacott (Conservative – Saskatoon-Wanuskewin) took the opportunity to note that preborn human children also feel pain, pain and suffering that is not recognized in Canadian law which allows for legal abortion through all nine months of a pregnancy.

On the floor of the House of Commons, Vellacott said:

Mr. Speaker, as a follow up to that series of petitions in respect of the pain that animals feel and in view of the fact that babies in the womb for the entire nine months feel some considerable pain caused by the abortion procedures that are used in this country, these petitioners in the country of Canada note that in the Canadian Charter of Rights and Freedoms everyone has a right to life, freedom from pain and freedom from the kind of assault fetuses experience in the womb.

It has been 47 years, since May 14, 1969, when Parliament changed the law to permit abortions and since January 28, 1988 Canada has had no law to protect the lives of unborn children. The petitioners are calling on Parliament, as the Supreme Court also urged, to pass legislation for the protection of human life from the time of conception and fertilization until the time of natural death.

The forty days for Life campaign to end Abortion.
We are the defenders of true freedom. May our witness unveil the deception of the "pro-choice" slogan.**Scripture:** Now the Lord is the Spirit; and where the Spirit of the Lord is, there is liberty.—2 Corinthians 3:17 Reflection: Norma McCorvey (the former Jane Roe of *Roe v. Wade*) used to work at an abortion mill named "A Choice for Women." She now realizes what a cruel irony that title was. She saw first hand, just as pregnancy resource center counselors see, that women don't get abortions because of freedom of choice, but rather because they feel they have no freedom and no choice. They feel trapped, abandoned, desperate and afraid, and have

been led to believe that abortion is their only option. As Frederica Mathewes-Green has written, no one wants an abortion like she wants a Porsche or an ice cream; rather, she wants it like an animal caught in a trap wants to gnaw off its own leg.

"Where the Spirit of the Lord is, there is liberty." That doesn't mean that the Spirit allows us to do whatever we want or to decide for ourselves what's right and wrong.Rather, it means that the Spirit gives us the freedom to do what is right, the power to choose what is good, when we see it before us and yet feel pulled in the opposite direction. Liberty means that we no longer have to feel doomed to do what we know is wrong. We are the people of the Spirit of the Lord, and when we take action on behalf of life, especially by being present at abortion mills, we are acting on behalf of true freedom, and imparting to those who are in bondage the power to do what is right.

Prayer: Come, Holy Spirit. You are the Spirit of freedom, the source of all that is good, the power to do what is right. Fill us, and fill those who are in bondage today, feeling doomed to do what is wrong. Set them free, and help us to hasten them on the road to freedom, where your grace overcomes every temptation. We ask this through Christ our Lord. Amen.
Fr. Frank Pavone
National Director, Priests for Life and President, National Pro-life Religious Council

"I Just Can't Take it Any More": Thanks to 40 Days for Life, Woman Wants Out of Abortion Business Commentary by Shawn Carney, Spring Campaign Director, 40 Days for LifeApril 1, 2009 (LifeSiteNews.com) - I won't tell you where this is happening, but there is a woman we know of who's pondering a career change. An abortion center employee has been talking to the 40 Days for Life prayer volunteers outside of her workplace - and she wants out! Her message was simple - she just couldn't take it any longer. It was time to look for a new job. She asked the vigil participants to pray for her. She said she couldn't simply quit her job, because she needs the income. Her prayer request was that she be able to find a suitable position elsewhere so she could give her notice at the clinic.She also said the prayers of the vigil participants have a definite impact at the clinic. "When there are prayers happening outside, she said the tone of what happens inside changes," the local campaign coordinator told me. "Everyone is aware of their presence, and she for one, can no longer pretend that what is happening is OK."

There are women in Carson City, Nevada who "can't take it any longer" either. Because of 40 Days for Life, they've learned the shocking truth that the ob/gyn practice they go to for routine health care also does abortions. It is indeed a fact that many people are simply unaware that abortions are going on in their own communities - even at their own doctors' offices. But thanks to vigil participants and pro-life supporters, 40 Days for Life is opening their eyes. This ob/gyn practice is "feeling the heat of our presence," said Carol Marie, one of the local 40 Days for Life coordinators. "We know of at least three patients who have left the practice once they learned that abortions are performed."

One of those women told the abortion clinic staff she would no longer be their patient and the receptionist gave her a stack of forms to fill out. But the woman's response was that she was only interested in one form - a form where she could explain to this medical practice why she was going away." She then proceeded to put a long note in writing as to exactly what she thought of an ob/gyn center performing abortions as a part of their regular practice," Carol Marie said. "This wonderful woman has ensured that they fully appreciate the reason they have lost her as a patient. By being present at the sidewalk, we are informing their patients about what is being done behind closed doors," she said. "With enough patients lost, they could rethink their commitment to performing abortions." She added, "If you ever wondered if what we've been doing has been making a difference, well the Lord has given us an answer, loud and clear.

Canada March for Life Marks 40 Years of Abortions, Pro-Life Group Seeks Debate

Ottawa, Canada (LifeNews.com) — Tens of thousands of Canadians mark 40 years of abortions in Canada. As pro-life advocates head to the nation's capital, the head of one pro-life group wonders why the Canadian parliament refuses to debate the issue. In May 1969, the Canadian government approved the passage of a bill that took off the books many of the protective laws the nation had in place. Then, in January 1988, the nation's abortion law was struck down from the Criminal Code by the Supreme Court of Canada resulting in full legal abortion on demand through all nine months of pregnancy. As a result, there have been more than 3.5 million abortions in Canada, resulting the death of babies before birth and injuring countless women. Michele Boulva, director of the Catholic Organization for Life and Family, is calling for a public debate on abortion. "Unlimited abortion has not gathered the support of a majority of Canadians, but it hangs on because of public indifference and silence, as well as a widespread lack of information about the full extent of Canada's juridical void on abortion, due in no small part to a silence on this topic by most media," she said. Full story at LifeNews.com

9. Homosexuality. Gay Sex is Downright Dangerous and Abstinence Won't Kill You: I Should Know

Commentary by David MacDonald

(Note: David MacDonald is a Christian singer/artist who recently revealed that prior to his conversion he had been heavily involved in the gay lifestyle. Read his testimony here: http://www.GayTestimony.com)March 10, 2009 (LifeSiteNews.com) - I hate to quote statistics, but Canada's largest gay paper XTRA recently reported that, "A group of six Canadian queers is taking on homophobia in Canada's healthcare system by filing a complaint with the Canadian Human Rights Commission."Gens Hellquist, one of the complainants, is the executive director of the Canadian Rainbow Health Coalition. She explained at length her concerns about the health status of homosexual men and women in Canada, observing: "We have one of the poorest health statuses in this country ... Health issues affecting queer Canadians includes lower life expectancy than the average Canadian, suicide, higher rates of substance abuse, depression, inadequate access to care and HIV/AIDS."

"There are all kinds of health issues that are endemic to our community," Hellquist continued. "We have higher rates of anal cancer in the gay male community, lesbians have higher rates of breast cancer ... the reality is there is (sic) more GLBT people in this country who die of suicide each year than die from AIDS, there are more who die early deaths from substance abuse than die of HIV/AIDS. ... Now that we can get married everyone assumes that we don't have any issues any more. A lot of the deaths that occur in our community are hidden, we don't see them. Those of us who are working on the front lines see them and I'm tired of watching my community die."

This seemed amazing to me, given that Hellquist appears to be arguing against the foundation of the gay rights movement. Now queer community leaders are admitting that gay sex is downright dangerous. But rather than speak about abstinence, they say they require the government to shift public health priorities away from the average population to the queer community, even though the statistics they provide demonstrate disproportionately higher spending on the gay community currently. Here are some of the stats that they cite in their human rights complaint:

• Life expectancy of gay/bisexual men in Canada is 20 years less than the average; that is 55 years.
• GLB people commit suicide at rates from 2 to 13.9 times more often than average.
• GLB people have smoking rates 1.3 to 3 times higher than average.

- GLB people have rates of alcoholism 1.4 to 7 times higher than average.
- GLB people have rates of illicit drug use 1.6 to 19 times higher than average.
- GLB people show rates of depression 1.8 to 3 times higher than average.
- Gay and bisexual men (MSM) comprise 76.1% of AIDS cases.
- Gay and bisexual men (MSM) comprise 54% of new HIV infections each year.If one uses Statistics Canada figure of 1.7% of GLB becoming infected, that is 26 times higher than average.GLB people are at a higher risk for anal cancers.Some gay activists say that the high levels of promiscuity and related STI's, partner abuse, addiction, and suicide in the gay community are because gay men have delayed adolescence as a result of "coming out" late (i.e., in their 30's), and they are promiscuous because they were late blooming teenagers. They say, "Does your gay age match your chronological age?"

If that theory was true then the statistics would show the promiscuity of adult gay men to be similar to straight teenagers. But adult gay men have promiscuity statistics far exceeding straight teenagers. The other problem with this theory is that there is no indication that the "adolescent sex craze" period slows down after 5 years of coming out, as it does after adolescents finish their teen years. In many cases the addiction to lust increases over time. Articles in gay papers frequently ridicule gay men who don't want exposure to HIV, and they encourage them to not curb sex. The culture of pushing sex down people's throats is not working. There is nothing wrong with abstinence from sex. This goes for everyone who is not married to someone of the opposite sex. I've been single and chaste for many years after having left the gay community. You don't die from not having sex. It's not like air or water.

Recent laws, policies and public funding aimed at reducing the rate of suicide, addiction, partner abuse, and STI's by granting more sexual freedom have not diminished those statistics. In fact, there has been an increase since the beginning of the 'rights' movement in the early 70's, and it's getting worse, not better. In places like San Francisco and the Netherlands where gay sex has been normalized, many of these stats are worse, so I have difficulty with the theory that more freedom, money and legislation will reduce these stats. That is just not where the facts point.The Church talks about Natural Law and says that if something is true it will prove true in many ways. The Bible says gay sex is a problem, biology doesn't support it, and health statistics demonstrate its problems. Why not abstain? That's what I'm doing. This is an excerpt of an article published here:

http://www.davidmacd.com/catholic/why_catholics_against_gay_sex.htm- DavidMacDonald's testimony about his time in the gay community is here: http://www.GayTestimony.com ;See related article: 14 Million See Italian Pop Star Sing of Victory over Homosexuality http://www.lifesitenews.com/ldn/2009/feb/09022014.html . In **May 2001 in Washington DC, CWNews.com ca /LSN.** reported the news that Dr Robert Spitzer, the instrumental figure in the 1973 decision of the American Psychiatric Association to remove homosexuality from its Diagnostic and Statistical manual of mental disorders , announced a new study which has altered his beliefs about the issue."I thought homosexual behavior could be resisted but sexual orientation could not be changed. I now believe that's untrue-some people can and do change."

10-May-2001 -- EWTN News Brief

NEW STUDY REVEALS HOMOSEXUALS CAN CHANGE

WASHINGTON, DC, (CWNews.com/LSN.ca) - Dr. Robert Spitzer, the instrumental figure in the American Psychiatric Association's 1973 decision to remove homosexuality from its diagnostic manual of mental disorders, has announced a new study, which has altered his beliefs on the issue.

"Like most psychiatrists," said Spitzer, "I thought that homosexual behavior could be resisted, but sexual orientation could not be changed. I now believe that's untrue-- some people can and do change." Spitzer presented his study on Wednesday at the annual meeting of the American Psychiatric Association.

In the most detailed investigation of sexual orientation change to date, Spitzer interviewed 200 subjects (143 men and 57 women) who had experienced a significant shift from homosexual to heterosexual attraction, which had lasted for at least five years. Most of the subjects said their religious faith was very important in their lives, and about three-quarters of the men and half of the women had been heterosexually married by the time of the study. Most had sought change because a gay lifestyle had been emotionally unsatisfying. Many had been disturbed by promiscuity, stormy relationships, a conflict with their religious values, and the desire to be (or to stay) heterosexually married.

Typically, the effort to change did not produce significant results for the first two years. Subjects said they were helped by examining their family and childhood experiences, and understanding how those factors might have contributed to their gender identity and sexual orientation. Same-sex mentoring relationships, behavior-therapy techniques, and group therapy were also mentioned as particularly helpful.

To the researchers' surprise, good heterosexual functioning was reportedly achieved by 67 percent of the men who had rarely or never felt any opposite-sex attraction before the change process. Nearly all the subjects said they now feel more masculine (in the case of men) or more feminine (women).

Spitzer concludes, "Contrary to conventional wisdom, some highly motivated individuals, using a variety of change efforts, can make substantial change in multiple indicators of sexual orientation, and achieve good heterosexual functioning." But, Spitzer said, his findings suggest that complete change-- cessation of all homosexual fantasies and attractions (which is generally considered an unrealistic goal in most therapies) is probably uncommon. Still, when subjects did not actually change sexual orientation-- for example, their change had been one of behavioral control and self-identity, but no significant shift in attractions-- they still reported an improvement in overall emotional health and functioning.

FEEL FREE TO SEND THIS TO COLLEAGUES AND TO POST THIS ON PROFESSIONAL LISTSERVES. THIS IS BEING SENT TO AUTHORS OF RECENT ARTICLES IN THE AMERICAN JOURNAL OF PSYCHIATRY, THE ARCHIVES OF GENERAL PSYCHIATRY AND THE JOURNAL OF ABNORMAL PSYCHOLOGY.

In my own specialty, psychiatry, back in 1973, the American Psychiatric Association, for purely political reasons and nothing to do with science, declared that homosexuality was no longer to be listed as a clinical abnormality. From then on all, even those who want treatment for homosexuality, can no longer expect to have their health insurance cover the cost of any treatment. Even though in the last few years a doctor who was a driving force in the 1972 decision, has since reversed his opinion based on his research findings, those who want to be treated and those who offer treatment, are still fighting, so far unsuccessfully, for the medical insurances to pay for treatments

9. Psychiatrists Revise Diagnostic Manual - In Secret

While we are on the subject of the DSM IV manual the number of categories of psychiatric "illnesses" from DSM 1 and II to DSM IV TR and soon DSM V has multiplied exponentially. All these new categories of psychiatric "illnesses " seem to only serve to complicate, not to simplify things in my opinion. (see below).

Robert L. Spitzer, M.D.
Professor of Psychiatry, Columbia University
Former Chair of Work Group to Develop DSM-III and DSM-III-R
Email address: Spitzer8@verizon.net

There is great interest in the development of DSM-V. Perhaps the best-kept-secret about DSM-V is that rather than being "an open and transparent process" as has been claimed by the American PsychiatricAssociation leadership (Rabinowitz, Psychiatric News, June 6 , 2008) it will essentially be developed in secret. This became apparent when Darrel Regier,Vice Chair and David Kupfer, Chair of the DSM-V revision, informed me that they would not let me have the minutes of DSM-V Task Force meetings, as I had repeatedly requested (Email Regier to Spitzer, February 23, 2008). They said this was because the Board of Trustees of the American Psychiatric Association believed it was "important to maintain DSM-V confidentiality."All DSM-V Task Force and Work Group members are therefore required to sign a"confidentiality agreement" which prohibits members from disclosing anything about DSM-V to anyone. The only exceptions are if the Task Force or Work Group member believes that the disclosure is "necessary for the development of DSM-V", the material has already been published by the APA or the DSM-V leadership has given permission for the disclosure.. Although the actual confidentiality agreement that members sign does not mention minutes of Task Force and Work Group meetings, the refusal of the DSM-V leadership to let me (or anyone else) have access to the minutes of DSM-V meetings is a logical consequence of the confidentiality agreements that all DSM-V members sign.

It should be noted that in contrast to this new APA confidentiality policy, which discourages DSM-V members from providing information about the ongoing revision process, the World Health Organization has adopted the opposite policy with regard to its development of ICD-11. Minutes of all ICD-11 meetings are posted on the WHO website without any restrictions on who can have access
http://www.who.int/mental_health/evidence/en/.

Ever since I became aware of this new DSM-V policy, I have tried to understand its justification and purpose by exchanging email letters with the APA and DSM-V leadership, and by an exchange of letters in Psychiatric News (Quotes in italic are from these letters which are all available on web site generously developed by Mike Miller http://taxa.epi.umn.edu/~mbmiller/sscpnet/20080909_Spitzer/According to the APA and DSM-V leadership, an important benefit of the confidentiality agreements is that it. "allows Task Force and Work Groupmembers to.freely discuss and candidly exchange their views with others in their Work Group or the DSM-V Task Force without concern that those initial and perhaps tentative views will be made public." This is ludicrous. It has never been seen with previous DSM revisions. It is hard to imagine a distinguished DSM-V researcher or clinician being reluctant to speak candidly because of such concerns. I have seen Task Force and Work Group members in previous revisions concerned that their contribution to the revision was not made public but never that is was.

The DSM-V confidentiality agreements ".protect APA rights." This is puzzling. APA owns the copyright to all DSM publications. What rights might be in jeopardy??" "The current confidentiality agreements are narrow and ensure the integrity of the process used to develop DSM-V"Narrow? Here is what it covers: I will not, during the term of this appointment or after, divulge, furnish or make accessible to anyone or use in any way .any Confidential Information. I understand that "Confidential Information" includes all Work Product, unpublished manuscripts and drafts and other pre-publication materials, group discussions, internal correspondence, information about the development process and any other written or unwritten information, in any form, that emanates from or relates to my work with the APA task force or work group.Another benefit of the confidentiality agreements.avoidsincomplete and inaccurate information from being disseminated and misused.Sure - but that can happen with the final official DSM-V. The solution is not secrecy but an effective public affairs committee that quickly responds to inaccurate or unfair accounts of DSM drafts..Why minutes of the work group are not being distributed outside the work groups .for a number of reasons that were recommended by ourattorney. No response to a request for one of the reasons. It should be noted that I never received an answer when I asked for example of problems with the development of DSM-III, DSM-III-R and DSM-V that the Confidentiality Agreements are designed to avoid.

I return to the beginning claim by the APA that the development of DSM-V is "transparent and open." The Merriam Webster's dictionary defines transparent as "characterized by visibility or accessibility of information" and this is how the term is commonly used. The APA has provided the names of all of the DSM-V committee members, as well as information about each member's financial relationships with the pharmaceutical industry. This information is available to anyone interested. Thus, it is accurate to characterize the "who are the members of the DSM-V committees" aspect of the DSM-V revision as being transparent. However, by not making minutes of meetings available to all but a relatively few DSM-V insiders, the DSM-Vrevision process - what is discussed, what options were considered, who supported a particular viewpoint - is largely opaque.

The DSM-V revision process could easily become transparent by simply putting the minutes of all meetings and conference calls on the DSM-V Website. Dr. Regier claims that posting minutes on the DSM-V Website would require APA to spend "an inordinate amount of time and energy dealing with every spontaneous response that someone might make to even considering certain diagnostic issues." Making the DSM-V process transparent by posting the minutes on a public web site, as the WHO does for the ICD-11 revision groups, does not obligate the APA to respond to "every spontaneousresponse"? How much time does it take to ignore a crackpot blog posting?

If in fact there is an increased need for staff support to deal with the consequences of transparency, that is money well spent. Another precedent here is the President's Council for Bioethics, which posts transcriptions of its meetings online:
http://www.bioethics.gov/transcripts/

Outside review of DSM-V should be ongoing and begin early in the revision process, not after all the decisions have been made. It is clear that the confidentiality agreements are limiting critical review of the DSM-V revision - and perhaps this is the true motivation for instituting this unprecedented new policy. Unfettered critical review by colleagues – a foundation of science - should be encouraged - not discouraged. A Task Force or Work Group meeting that properly has a scientific discussion that is focused on methodological, empirical and practical issues should have nothing to hide from the public. It is ironic that one of the most widespread (and in my view unfair) criticisms of DSM-III and progeny has been the process of decision-making by committee. This silly new "confidentiality" policy plays right into the hands of these critics and fuels cynicism about the decision-making process - except that in this case, in contrast to decision making for the revision of prior DSMs, the cynicism may be well justified. The Board of Trustees of the APA will only reconsider this new policy if large numbers of mental health professionals protest the new policy and demand that the minutes of regular conference calls and meeting be made available to anyone interested.

With the help of Scott Lilienfeld and Jerry Rosen (psychologists), John

Sadler (psychiatrist) and Jerome Wakefield (social worker) an online petition will be developed (with Mike Miller's help) that will call on the American Psychiatric Association's Board of Trustees to open the DSM-V revision process by placing minutes of Task Force and Work Group conference calls and meetings on the DSM-V website.

Robert L. Spitzer, M.D.
Professor of Psychiatry
New York State Psychiatric Institute
Unit 60 —-1051 Riverside Drive
New York City, NY, 10533
Cell phone: 914-500-7941
Email: Spitzer8@Verizon.net

NY's Highest Court to Hear Appeal in Suits against Officials Who Attempted to Recognize Same-Sex "Marriage"

ALBANY, N.Y., April 1, 2009 (LifeSiteNews.com) - The New York Court of Appeals, the state's highest court, agreed Tuesday to hear two appeals filed by attorneys with the Alliance Defense Fund in lawsuits against officials who have attempted to recognize out-of-state same-sex "marriages" in contradiction to state law. "New York state and local officials shouldn't recognize the laws of foreign jurisdictions when they conflict with state law," said ADF Senior Legal Counsel Brian Raum. "These officials have overstepped their authority in order to forward the agenda of special interest groups."

ADF attorneys are arguing in Lewis v. New York State Department of Civil Service that the department illegally redefined the term "spouse" in order to extend marriage benefits to same-sex couples "wed" outside the state. On behalf of New York taxpayers, ADF attorneys filed the suit in May 2007, arguing that the directive illegally replaces state law with laws from foreign jurisdictions at the expense of taxpayers and families who have not consented to it. In Godfrey v. Spano, ADF attorneys argue that Westchester County Executive Andrew Spano illegally ordered county agencies to recognize out-of-state same-sex "marriages." In August 2006, ADF attorneys filed the suit to stop Spano from exceeding his constitutional authority. ADF-allied attorney Jim Trainor is serving as local counsel on the Lewis v. New York State Department of Civil Service case.

Change Is Possible for Gays, Says Psychologist
APA Admits Homosexuality Also Due to Environmental Factors   By Genevieve Pollock

ENCINO, California, JUNE 15, 2009 (Zenit.org).- A Catholic psychologist who specializes in reparative therapy with homosexuals says it's possible for those with same-sex attractions to change, despite agenda-driven ideologies that state the opposite.

Joseph Nicolosi, founder and director of the Thomas Aquinas Psychological Clinic in Encino, spoke with ZENIT about his experience as a clinical psychologist and the former president of the National Association for Research and Therapy of Homosexuality (NARTH).

NARTH, a "scientific, non-religious and non-political" organization, recently put out an article about the little known revision of the American Psychological Association's (APA) statement on homosexuality, which was highlighted last month in a WorldNetDaily article titled "Gay Gene Claim Suddenly Vanishes." Nicolosi explained that NARTH has been actively working on a research project compiling scientific data to dispute the APA's claim on homosexuality, targeting three unscientific assumptions that form the basis of their policy. He stated that these erroneous assumptions are: "Psychotherapy does not change homosexuality, trying to change the homosexual person will harm him, and there is no greater pathology in homosexual persons than in heterosexual persons."

The psychologist asserted that the "APA is not governed by scientists, but by political interests."

"There has been no new data to justify their policies," he added, "but they tend to give in to social and political pressure," and thus "NARTH has been putting pressure on them to scientifically back up their stance on the biological nature of homosexuality." Now, Nicolosi reported, the APA has "diminished its position saying homosexuality is biologically determined." They have dropped the specific reference to a hypothetical "gay gene," he affirmed. In other words, he said, they are beginning to recognize that homosexuality is also due to environmental factors, not just biological elements. "In fact," he stated, "I and many of my colleagues at NARTH believe it is more environmental than biological."

Nicolosi noted that "the most important scientific information" gives "much more evidence for environmental causes of homosexuality than for biological."

Possible

The most essential point however, the psychologist affirmed, "is that change is possible, that men and women can come out of homosexuality." This idea of 'once gay, always gay' is a political position, not a scientific position," he added.The therapist affirmed that he has seen this in his own private practice, and that it is also substantiated in a body of scientific research. Nicolosi, also the author of "Healing Homosexuality: Case Stories of Reparative Therapy" and "A Parent's Guide to Preventing Homosexuality," asserted that many people have already adopted the erroneous assumptions put forth by the APA.

There is a need to assist and minister to men and women "who are looking for help to come out of homosexuality," he said, "because so many times they are just told 'Well, you're born this way,' pointing to the APA and saying 'because they said it.'"He expressed the hope that as the APA recognizes the efficacy of therapy with homosexual persons, more psychologists will be encouraged to be involved in this type of treatment." Within our profession," the psychologist explained, "we trump politics with science." In other words, if we challenge the APA with scientific data, it "has to override any political or special interest forces." The therapist emphasized the need for all people to share this message with homosexual persons that "you don't have to be gay."

Encouragement

If you know a homosexual person, he said, "encourage that person, educate him, give that person information, take the opportunity to let him know that choice is possible." "They need to believe it," he added. Nicolosi explained: "It is a very hard therapy. First of all, it is hard in itself because you have to dig deep into emotional issues. Homosexuality is not about sexual issues, but emotional. There are the emotional underpinnings that have to be addressed." Then not only are you having to deal with those emotional underpinnings that are challenging on an individual level, but you have the other battle of a culture that is saying to you, 'You're homophobic; you're naïve; you're not facing reality; you're just a guilt-ridden Christian, get with it

"You're fighting a culture that is not supporting you, plus you have your own individual battle. So it's a two-front war." "With the AIDS epidemic, this could be about life and death here," he asserted. "We're not talking about something insignificant ."The psychologist underlined the need to "inform and educate young people." He explained: "So when a 15-year-old boy goes to a priest and says, 'Father I have these feelings, I have these temptations,' that priest should say, 'you have a choice; if you don't want to be gay there are things that you can do.'"

"The boy should not to be told, 'God made you this way,'" Nicolosi said.

Scientific data

He continued: "This is not about going after an oppressed minority. It's not about pointing out pathology for the sake of pointing out pathology." This is telling young people, look, if you go down this road, you are likely to have a higher level of depression, anxiety, failed relationships, sexual promiscuity, drug and alcohol abuse than people who live their lives heterosexually. You will get involved in more, to be polite, esoteric exotic sexual practices. It goes on and on and on. "And that's just science, simply a comparison of two groups."

The therapist added, "This notion that you are going to fall in love with a man and live happily ever after is Hollywood. The reality is that it's a hard lifestyle." Nicolosi, also a national speaker on the topic, urged the development of more Catholic programs, noting that other faiths have already been putting forth a "vital ministry helping people coming out of homosexuality." "Our doctrine is clear," he said, "and even if we have a weaker ministry, our doctrine on homosexuality is more brilliant than anything the Protestant denominations can come up with."

The psychologist specifically referenced a 1986 document signed by Cardinal Joseph Ratzinger before he became Pope, addressed to the Catholic bishops "On the Pastoral Care of Homosexual Persons." In the letter, the cardinal, at that time prefect of the Congregation for the Doctrine of the Faith, outlined the moral underpinnings and practical considerations of the pastoral care of "those whose suffering can only be intensified by error and lightened by truth."

In this light, Nicolosi underlined the importance of helping homosexual persons who want to change, because "if you are Christian, you have to believe that you are intended for the opposite sex" and that "sexual complementarity is part of the natural law."

This is something that "should be evident to everyone," as "our Christian anthropology," he stated, and yet "it is amazing" how many people are confused about this." They actually believe, or want to believe, either for personal reasons or political reasons, that God created two kinds of people: homosexuals and heterosexuals," Nicolosi noted."It is seeping into the consciousness without critical evaluation," he cautioned, the resignation that "God just made them that way."

Courage

The psychologist appealed to priests to not be intimidated to teach about homosexuality from the pulpit, noting that he has met many Catholics who are "discouraged that there is no resource for them." "We have Courage as the only orthodox Catholic ministry, and it's underfunded, underrepresented and essentially pushed to the side," he stated. He reported that "Courage is only represented in 10% of the parishes in this country" and thus many "men and women who want to come out of homosexuality" are left without resources on a local level, making it "very tough for them." Nicolosi suggested that if a priest is working with a homosexual person and is uncertain about how to help, to refer him to a reparative therapist, "who really knows about this particular kind of treatment."

"Not to just any generic psychotherapist," he added, "but to a therapist who has training in sexual re-orientation change." Referencing Cardinal Ratzinger's letter, he warned against a "studied ambiguity" in the face of the real need homosexual persons have for outreach from the Church.

On the Net:

National Association for Research and Therapy of Homosexuality Web site:www.narth.com
Cardinal Ratzinger's Letter:
http://www.vatican.va/roman_curia/congregations/cfaith/documents/rc_co n_cfaith_doc_19861001_homosexual-persons_en.html email this article | print this article | comment this article

APA Officially Rejects Reorientation Treatment for HomosexualsOverwhelming research from the past hundred years rejected due to "serious design flaws." By Patrick B. Craine

August 5, 2009 (LifeSiteNews.com) - The American Psychological Association (APA) adopted a resolution Wednesday urging mental health professionals to avoid telling clients that they can change their sexual orientation through therapy or other treatments. The decision rejects the hundred years' worth of research indicating the effectiveness and benefits of sexual reorientation therapy due to "serious design flaws." The resolution also advises that parents, guardians, young people and their families avoid sexual orientation treatments that portray homosexuality as a mental illness and rather seek treatments "that provide accurate information on sexual orientation and sexuality, increase family and school support and reduce rejection of sexual minority youth." The approval was made at the APA's annual convention with a 125-4 vote. At the convention, a task force presented a report that in part examined the efficacy of 'reparative therapy,' or sexual orientation change efforts (SOCE). The task force examined the

83 studies conducted in English between 1960 and 2007 regarding SOCE, but concluded that the vast majority of the studies were unacceptable because of poor methodology. "Unfortunately, much of the research in the area of sexual orientation change contains serious design flaws," task force chair Dr. Judith M. Glassgold said. "Few studies could be considered methodologically sound and none systematically evaluated potential harms."

Dr. Joseph Nicolosi, founder and director of the Thomas Aquinas Psychological Clinic, disagreed, according to CitizenLink. Nicolosi claims the organization did not give sufficient weight to the years of clinical research that shows that in some cases sexual orientation is changeable through therapy. "The APA is really failing to not only represent science, which is its primary responsibility," he said, "but it's also failing to inform people." While not making a definitive statement, the task force suggested that SOCE carried a potential for harm. "There are no methodologically sound studies of recent SOCE that would enable the task force to make a definitive statement about whether or not recent SOCE is safe or harmful and for whom," the report says. Elaborating, Glassgold said, "Without such information, psychologists cannot predict the impact of these treatments and need to be very cautious, given that some qualitative research suggests the potential for harm."

Reiterating the APA stance that homosexuality is not a mental disorder, a decision made in 1973, the report cites the work of Dr. Evelyn Hooker. Hooker's research purportedly showed that pathology was no more apparent in homosexuals than in heterosexuals. Though her work has been harshly criticized, and is effectively debunked, Hooker is considered by some to be the mother of the homosexual movement, and her 1957 study was one of two cited in the 1973 decision. The purpose of her 1957 study was to analyze the prevalence of mental instability in homosexuals by comparing a group of homosexual men with a group of heterosexual men. The study's homosexual subjects, however, were screened and selected by the Mattachine Society, a newly-formed homosexual activist organization, who removed individuals from the homosexual group who showed signs of mental instability. According to Jeff Johnston, gender issues analyst for Focus on the Family, the APA has based its guidelines on the false premise that homosexuality is normal and positive. "There are a lot of people out there who haven't just changed their sexual identity or behavior, but their attractions have also changed," he told CitizenLink. "I'm one of those people."

In fact, the task force report accepts the normality of homosexual behaviour without question, and begins its resolution with that premise, citing as evidence, most notably, the 1948 and 1953 studies of Alfred Kinsey. The research of Kinsey, however, considered the father of the sexual revolution, has been discredited by Dr. Judith Reisman, who revealed in her book "Kinsey: Crimes and Consequences," that his survey populations were substantially drawn from prison inmates and homosexual bars, though he represented them as indicative of the general population. With such support, the APA declares: "Be it resolved, That the American Psychological Association affirms that same-sex sexual and romantic attractions, feelings, and behaviors are normal and positive variations of human sexuality regardless of sexual orientation identity."

The report also addressed the potential for conflict between one's religious faith and homosexual orientation, with many seeking a change in sexual orientation due to a conflict with their beliefs. The task force recommended that mental health practitioners help clients "explore possible life paths that address the reality of their sexual orientation, reduce the stigma associated with homosexuality, respect the client's religious beliefs, and consider possibilities for a religiously and spiritually meaningful and rewarding life." "In other words," Glassgold said, "we recommend that psychologists be completely honest about the likelihood of sexual orientation change, and that they help clients explore their assumptions and goals with respect to both religion and sexuality."

The National Association for Research and Therapy of Homosexuality (NARTH) refuted the APA's claims in a meta-analysis they issued in their Journal of Human Sexuality. They showed that over 100 years of research indicates that treatment for unwanted homosexuality can be beneficial. According to their analysis of the research, reparative therapy is effective and is generally not harmful. They demonstrate, further, that pathology has been found to be significantly greater in the homosexual community. In a press release issued today, NARTH Vice-President of Operations David Pruden expressed appreciation for the APA's recognition of the importance of faith and religious diversity, but accused the organization of bias in its selection of the task force.

"The task force reflected virtually no ideological diversity," he says. "No APA member who offers reorientation therapy was allowed to join the task force. In fact, one can make the case that every member of the task force can be classified as an activist.

"They selected and interpreted studies that fit within their innate and immutable view," he continues, pointing out two key studies that they omitted, and one that they downplayed. "Had the task force been more neutral in their approach, they could have arrived at only one conclusion: homosexuality is not invariable fixed in all people, and some people can and do change, not just in terms of behavior and identity but in core features of sexual orientation such as fantasy and attractions." Regarding the potential for harm associated with treatment, "as in all provisions of psychological care, the possibility exists that the client may not be happy with the outcome," Pruden comments. "Further, if some clients are dissatisfied with the therapeutic outcome, as in therapy for other issues, the possibility for dissatisfaction appears to be outweighed by the potential gains. The possibility of dissatisfaction also seems insignificant when compared to the substantial medical, emotional, and physical risks associated with homosexual behavior."

"NARTH would suggest that these medical and emotional risks," he concludes, "along with the incongruity of homosexual behavior with the personal and religious values of many people will continue to be the motivation for some individuals to seek assistance for their unwanted homosexual attraction." See related LifeSiteNews.com coverage:

16-Jul-2001 -- ZENIT.org News Agency
ZENIT material may not be reproduced without permission. Permission can be requested at info@zenit.org

BIBLE CITATIONS ADD UP TO HATE SPEECH, PANEL SAYS

Christian Ordered to Pay Activists Over Newspaper

SASKATOON, Saskatchewan, (Zenit.org).- What do Romans 1, Leviticus 18:22 and 20:13, and 1 Corinthians 6:9-10 have in common?

References to them can be "hate speech," says the Canadian province of Saskatchewan's Human Rights Commission.

In a ruling last month, the commission ordered both the Saskatoon StarPhoenix newspaper and Hugh Owens of Regina to pay $1,500 to three homosexual activists for publishing an advertisement with the references to four biblical verses condemning homosexuality, the National Catholic Register reported.

The ruling also bars Owens from "further publishing or displaying the bumper stickers" upon which his newspaper advertisement was based, according to the Register.

On June 30, 1997, Owens placed an advertisement in the StarPhoenix, on the occasion of Saskatoon's Homosexual Pride Week. His ad listed four Bible references followed by an equal sign and the universal prohibition sign -- a circle with a slash -- containing two stick-men holding hands.

In its decision against Owens and the StarPhoenix, the human rights commission judged that, "while the stick-figures are more neutral," it is the "combination of the prohibition symbol with the Bible passages that exposes homosexuals to hatred."

The three homosexual activists had filed a complaint with the human rights commission, noting that provincial and federal human rights codes both include "sexual orientation" as a protected category.

The commission ruled that the provincial human rights code can place "reasonable restriction" on Owen's religious expression, since the advertisement exposed the complainants "to hatred, ridicule, and their dignity was affronted on the basis of their sexual orientation."

Father Paul Donlevy, vicar general for the Diocese of Saskatoon, testified before the panel that the Catholic Church understands sexual orientation may not be chosen, but nevertheless "every person is called to holiness ... and homosexuals are called to the same sexual morality as any other unmarried people."

Mega Analysis of Over 100 Years of Research Shows Treatment for Unwanted Homosexuality Beneficial http://www.lifesitenews.com/ldn/2009/jun/09062309.html
Kinsey: Crime of the Century http://www.lifesitenews.com/ldn/1999/jan/99012803.html
The Mother of the Homosexual Movement - Evelyn Hooker PhD http://www.lifesitenews.com/ldn/2007/jul/07071603.html

In recent months I have been hearing documentaries stating that the amount of oestrogen products, derived from plastic food wrappings and being seen in the environment in the waters, is having a significant influence on the feminizing of animals as well as boys being born.

Web Search Results 1-10 of about **141** for **Oestrogen in the environment feminizing...**

Boys Will Be Girls - Health News

boys will be girls, pseudo-estrogens in plastics, in food packaging, ... of feminized human males as yet, there are other, more subtle signs that we are being affected as well. Homosexual orientation and a tendency towards obesity They can mimic the female hormone oestrogen when ingested. ...www.truehealth.org/ahealn41.html

also search CBC news /sperm count reduction /fewer male babies being born/ plastic food wrappings discarded contaminating water producing oestrogen-like hormones /effect on males.

10. Brain Death and Organ Donation.

In the great flurry to get organs, in these times, we don't seem to stop and wonder why, after all these centuries, there is such an insatiable need for organs in this and last century when this was not so in previous centuries.

What about the fact that in every nation at all previous times, the ordinary man in the street could nearly always tell when another human being was dead by universally recognizable cardio-pulmonary criteria. Now the diagnosis "brain death," is only recognized(diagnosable) by a select few doctors while the poor relatives looking on (if allowed since there is a movement that believes relatives should not have a say and should not even be allowed to participate in the decision)see their relative pink and warm but declared "brain dead."

It is not only the fact that they may often be killing someone whose soul is still present, but there is also the issue that they may be ignoring the fact that they are taking the life of someone whom God is not calling Home yet, and prolonging a life that He may be calling Home! I have met surgeons who no longer perform transplantations because they have this very concern—- "killing those who aught not to die; keeping alive those who aught not to live: lying to my people who love to hear lies." Ezekiel [13:19]. . God, not limited by time, utters Words that can apply through all times!

The President's Council on Bioethics paper *is a recent, balanced though not all-inclusive document on the subject of brain death chaired by Dr Edmund Pellegrino, Professor of Medicine and Ethics at Georgetown. It is well worth reading and I have provided the reference for anyone interested in the whole paper.*

Controversies in the Determination of Death: A White Paper by the President's Council on Bioethics, The President's Council on Bioethics. Washington, DC: January 2009. Available online at: www.bioethics.gov/reports/death/index.html.

It is worth noting that in the end the consensus was in favour of brain death but it was not unanimous. Dr Pellegrino was the chairman of the council and also one of the dissenters and a faithful Catholic. His paper at the end spells out his reasons for dissenting very clearly and I am quoting the last two paragraphs in particular because the last sentence is also both the "gold standard" on the diagnosis of death as well as the Roman Catholic Church's position on the subject of death.

Dr Pellegrino's Quote

"Ultimately, the central ethical challenge for any transplantation protocol is to give the gift of life to one human being without taking life away from another. Until the uncertainties and imprecision of the life-death spectrum so clearly recognized by Hans Jonas are dispelled, his moral advice must be our guide for all transplant protocols: We do not know with certainty the borderline between life and death, and a definition cannot substitute for knowledge.

Moreover, we have sufficient grounds for suspecting that the artificially supported condition of the comatose patient may still be one of life, however reduced—i.e., for doubting that, even with the brain function gone, he is completely dead. In this state of marginal ignorance and doubt the only course to take is to lean over backward toward the side of possible life."

It is also worth noting that both our present Holy Father, Pope Benedict XVI and John-Paul II, in their respective addresses to the transplant community specified their wish that the WHOLE scientific community reach agreement on the issue of brain death, (the neurological definition of death;) both popes are being ignored by and large.

But here even the best of the best could not agree. Furthermore, in all this juggling with strategies to find the fastest way to reap the organs, as seen below and in reading Dr Pellegrino's last paragraph we Christians should not lose sight of the fact that we do not know for certain when the soul of the donor has been called home by God.

Much more could be said on this subject but I will quote my friend Nancy Valko with her consent, who summarized the contents of the white paper very well.

Death and the Organ Donor by Nancy Valko, RN

In the early 1970s, I was a young nurse working with many trauma victims in a state-of-the-art intensive care unit and I loved it. Because of the high number of young accident victims, I was also often involved with organ donation from patients diagnosed as brain-dead. Asking shocked and grieving relatives about organ donation was the hardest part of my work.

Back then, "brain death" was a new legal and ethical concept stemming from an influential 1968 Harvard medical school committee paper titled "A Definition of Irreversible Coma", which concluded that severely brain-injured patients who met certain criteria could be pronounced dead before the heart stops beating. Starting in the early 1970s, various state legislatures and courts acted to turn this "medical consensus" into a legally recognized standard for determining death by loss of all brain function. Patients declared "brain-dead" then could have their organs harvested while their hearts were still beating and a ventilator kept their lungs going. The brain death concept virtually created the modern transplant system because waiting to take organs until breathing and heartbeat naturally stopped usually resulted in unusable, damaged vital organs.

Like most people, I didn't know the history of brain death back then and despite the tragic circumstances of my "brain- dead" patients, I was excited by the opportunity to participate in turning tragedy into the "gift of life".

Over time, however, I developed some nagging concerns about the brain-death concept and I shared them with our intensive care doctors. I was told, as one doctor put it, "Nancy, greater minds than yours have already figured this all out so don't worry about it." It took me years to realize that this meant these doctors didn't know the answers either.

Death and Choice Unknown to most people, controversy about brain death has simmered for years in the bioethics community. Some well-known physicians, for example, Alan Shewmon and Paul Byrne, argue that the current brain-death standard does not reflect true death. Others, such as Dr. Ron Cranford and ethicist Robert Veatch, argue that the brain-death standard should be stretched to include so-called "persistent vegetative" patients, further expanding the pool of potential organ donors.

Last August the bioethics world was rocked by an article by Drs. Robert Truog and Franklin G. Miller in the prestigious New England Journal of Medicine that made the shocking assertion that many organ donors were not really dead at the time their vital organs were harvested.**1** This Harvard doctor and this National Institutes of Health bioethicist then proposed the radical idea that doctors should drop the rule requiring that people be declared dead before vital organs are taken in favor of merely "obtaining valid informed consent for organ donation from patients or surrogates before the withdrawal of life-sustaining treatment in situations of devastating and irreversible neurologic injury". This, in Truog's and Miller's opinion, would preserve the current transplant system and still be acceptable to the public because "issues related to respect for valid consent and the degree of neurologic injury may be more important to the public than concerns about whether the patient is already dead at the time organs are removed." Perhaps as a result of articles like this, the President's Council on Bioethics decided to explore the determination-of- death issues involved in organ transplantation. In January 2009, the Council published "Controversies in the Determination of Death: A White Paper".**2** Many of the report's consensus conclusions were surprising and controversial themselves.

The President's Council on Bioethics White Paper

The President's Council on Bioethics white paper on the determinations of death made several startling admissions, including finding that some of the most fundamental rationales for brain death were wrong. The Council, citing scientific studies and observations, admitted that the brain is apparently *not* the central organizing agent without which the body cannot function for more than a short period of time. Years ago, many of us questioned why some supposedly brain-dead pregnant women could be maintained on ventilators — for even up to a couple of months in some cases — in order to help their unborn children develop and survive birth. Others observed that some supposedly brain- dead children could actually grow and even sexually mature if maintained on life support. It turns out that we were right to question this allegedly settled matter.

The Council also had to admit the little-known fact that brain-death tests vary widely from institution to institution, potentially leading to people who could be declared brain-dead at one hospital but at a different hospital still be considered alive. Personally, I was disappointed that the Council's paper did not even mention instances like the recent Zach Dunlap case, in which every supposedly definitive brain-death test was done, but a last-minute response by Zach stopped the impending organ donation and Zach even recovered.[3]

But in the consensus opinion of the Council members, apparently the concept of brain death is just too big to fail. Accordingly, some members of the Council proposed that the term "brain death" be replaced with the term "total brain failure". And with the new term, these members created a new justification for harvesting the organs of people declared to have this condition. According to this redefinition, the brain is important not because it controls physiological processes, but because these processes represent "engagement with the world".

This "engagement with the world" takes three forms: openness to the world, an ability to act on the world, and the need to do so. These abstract requirements can be met by something as basic as breathing but they are not met by physiological activities that continue in people who have allegedly lost all neurological function. This, the Council members insisted, is enough to spare breathing, brain-injured people like Terri Schiavo from a diagnosis of "total brain failure". Ironically though, this assertion does not protect people like Terri from having vital organs removed during the time when they are initially placed on a ventilator because doctors can then use another, newer determination of death called "donation after cardiac death" or DCD (formerly known as "non-heartbeating organ donation" or NHBD).[4] The Council's white paper also addresses this type of death determination and, in the process, makes more startling admissions.

DCD/NHBD was developed in the early 1990s to promote a newer standard of determining death for the purpose of organ donation. DCD/NHBD describes a procedure in which a person is declared hopelessly brain-injured or ill but not brain-dead and, with the consent of the patient or surrogates (or potentially even a "living will"-style document), has his or her ventilator removed with the expectation that breathing and heartbeat will stop within about 1 hour. When the heartbeat and breathing stop for usually about 2 to 5 minutes, the person is declared dead and the organs are taken for transplant. If the person's heartbeat and breathing do not stop within the allotted time, the transplant is called off and the person is left to die without further treatment.

The Council's white paper admitted that the legal definition of *irreversible* cessation of heartbeat and breathing used to justify DCD/NHBD has problems. Most people would consider "irreversible" in this context to mean that the heart has lost the ability to beat. But in DCD/NHBD, "irreversible" instead means that there is a deliberate decision not to try to restart the heart when it stops and that enough time has elapsed to ensure that the heart will not resume beating on its own. However the Council had to admit the dearth of scientific evidence supporting this determination. In some cases involving babies, for instance, the heart is harvested and actually restarted in another baby.

The Council also admitted that even fully conscious but spinal-cord-injured patients have become DCD/NHBD donors when dependent on a ventilator. This sad fact is the result of virtually all withdrawal-of-treatment decisions now being considered legal and thus ethical. The Council also noted that even though doctors are advised to take their time determining death when a natural death occurs, the interval between declaring death and starting transplantation in a DCD/NHBD patient has been as short as 75 seconds. It seems obvious that the push for a speedy declaration of death is not about new scientific information determining the moment of death but rather a desire to quickly get organs because "[t]he longer a patient removed from ventilation 'lingers' before expiring, the more likely are the organs destined for transplantation to be damaged by warm ischemia [lack of adequate blood flow]".[5] But even while expressing concerns, the Council still supported the DCD/NHBD concept in the end.

Despite pages discussing these DCD/NHBD issues, the Council unfortunately ignored a most crucial issue: How do doctors determine who is a "hopeless enough" patient with functioning vital organs and who will also die fast enough to get usable organs? The Council never mentioned articles like the one in the September/October 2008 issue of the *Journal of Intensive*

Care Medicine, which stated "Donation failure [patients who don't die fast enough to have usable organs] has been reported in at least 20% of patients enrolled in DCD". Those authors also concluded that "There is little evidence to support that the DCD practice complies with the dead donor rule".6

We Are All Affected

While organ donation is a worthy goal when conducted ethically, it is very dangerous when physicians and ethicists redefine terms and devise new rationales without the knowledge or input of others, especially the public. This has been happening far too often and far too long in many areas of medical ethics and the consequences are often lethal. Opinions about medical ethics affect all of us and our loved ones. And good medical ethics decisions are the foundation of a trustworthy medical system. We are constantly exhorted to sign organ-donor cards and join state organ registries but are we getting enough accurate information to give our truly informed consent? This question is too important to just leave to the self-described experts.

Notes

1 "The Dead Donor Rule and Organ Transplantation", R. D. Truog and F. G. Miller. *New England Journal of Medicine*, August 14, 2008.

2 *Controversies in the Determination of Death: A White Paper by the President's Council on Bioethics*, The President's Council on Bioethics. Washington, DC: January 2009. Available online at: www.bioethics.gov/reports/death/index.html.

3 "Was Zach Dunlap's Recovery a Miracle?", Nancy Valko, RN. *Voices* Vol. XXIII, No. 2, Pentecost 2008. Available online at www.wf-f.org/08-2-Valko.html.

4 "Non-heart beating organ donation and the vegetative state", George Isajiw, MD and Nancy Valko, RN. March 2004. Available online at www.wf-f.org/NHBD-VatMar2004.html.

5 *Controversies in the Determination of Death: A White Paper by the President's Council on Bioethics*, page 82.

6 "Organ Procurement after Cardiocirculatory Death: A Critical Analysis", Mohamed Y. Rady, MD, PhD, Joseph L. Verheijde, PhD, MBA, and Joan McGregor, PhD. *Journal of Intensive Care Medicine*. September/October 2008, available online at http://jic.sagepub.com/cgi/reprint/23/5/303.pdf.

Nancy Valko, a registered nurse from St. Louis, is president of Missouri Nurses for Life, a spokesperson for the National Association of Pro-Life Nurses and a *Voices* contributing editor.

Consciousness, Coma, and Brain Death—2009
http://jama.ama-assn.org/cgi/content/full/301/11/1172

Comment: Note this quote: "a patient in PVS who appears unaware of the environment and commands actually may be fully aware and cognitively intact but unable to show any response to stimuli." Although this commentary accepts brain death criteria uncritically, it does give a good review of some new (and not so new) advances in understanding that lack of motion in brain injury does not automatically mean lack of brain function. I wish this had come out during Terri's ordeal and I doubt that this will come out in the mainstream media even now due to the medical, legal and public bias against people with severe brain injury.
Nancy V.

JAMA. 2009;301(11):1172-1174. With Commentary by Roger N. Rosenberg, MD following.

SUMMARY OF THE ORIGINAL ARTICLE
A Definition of Irreversible Coma: Report of the Ad Hoc Committee of the Harvard Medical School to Examine the Definition of Brain Death

Ad Hoc Committee of the Harvard Medical School to Examine the Definition of Brain Death
JAMA. 1968;205(6):337-340.

This landmark classic article was the first to quantitatively define the clinical and laboratory criteria used to measure the presence of brain death. The study included "only those comatose individuals who have no discernible central nervous system activity." Criteria to establish the presence of irreversible coma included (1) unreceptivity and unresponsitivity; (2) no movements or breathing; (3) no reflexes (brain stem); and (4) flat electroencephalogram. These criteria are still considered to be reliable and acceptable by the medical community and have become established into law, which states that brain death is equivalent to death and that all artificial support systems sustaining heart, respiratory, and metabolic functions can be legally stopped.
See PDF for full text of the original *JAMA* article.

Commentary

Coma refers to the clinical state in which a patient is unarousable and does not respond to stimuli. It may be caused by structural lesions to the brainstem, the thalamus, or the cerebral hemispheres, and by metabolic abnormalities.

Coma must be differentiated from the stuporous state in which the patient is unresponsive but with stimuli shows some evoked activity.[1] It must be distinguished from the persistent vegetative state (PVS),[2] a syndrome with several causes in which the patient has sustained severe brain damage, and in which coma has advanced to a state of wakefulness without detectable awareness. In addition, the minimal conscious state[3] has been described in which the patient exhibits definite responsiveness that is cognitively driven, rather than unconscious reflexive responses. There may be a progressive improving continuum from coma to PVS and then to minimal conscious state. The continuum can also proceed in an adverse manner with deterioration from coma to brain death, an irreversible clinical condition in which, by neurological examination, the patient has lost all brain stem reflexes, including any respiratory response to hypercapnea exceeding an arterial $PaCO_2$ of 60 mm Hg; and has normal routine clinical chemistry results, negative toxicology screen, normal body temperature, and absence of brain blood flow by diagnostic imaging procedures.[4]

Today neurologists routinely assess patients with impaired consciousness by performing a complete neurological examination to determine if the patient is stuporous, comatose, in PVS, or in a minimal conscious state. The challenge is then to determine if the basis for the altered level of consciousness is due to a structural lesion such as an infarction, hemorrhage, tumor, infection in the brain stem, thalamus, or cerebral hemispheres; or alternatively, due to a metabolic cause such as severe hypoglycemia, electrolyte disturbance, toxin or drug overdose. The neurological examination is crucial for determining the neuroanatomical level of the cause for evaluating whether there are specific brain stem signs such as cranial nerve defects, altered patterns of respiration, the presence of hemiplegia in relation to any cranial nerve deficits, and the occurrence of focal seizures such as myoclonus or focal motor seizures. Additional causes, including herniation syndromes (transtentorial, uncal, and cerebellar), are identifiable through a careful and thorough neurological examination.[1]

Coma as a clinical state has ancient roots, but the identification and precise codification of specific clinical neurological criteria for brain death causal of irreversible coma was first published in a now classic article in *JAMA* in 1968.[5] The criteria for brain death enumerated in this article have surely held up during the past 40 years. As reviewed by Joynt in 1984,[6] the Harvard criteria, as defined in the classic article for brain death, subsequently has had far-reaching positive consequences. The review[6] pointed out the potential clinical circumstance, a disparity that has been well documented, that a patient may have a dead brain in an otherwise healthy body and second, identification of an irreversible state of coma has made possible the ethical and practical donation of living organs from patients with brain death. The Uniform Determination of Death Act (http://www.hhs.gov/ohrp/documents/19830728.pdf) presented to President Reagan in 1981 stated: "An individual who has sustained either (1) irreversible cessation of circulatory and respiratory functions, or (2) irreversible cessation of all functions of the entire brain, including the brain stem, is dead." The denotation of a patient with brain death has become equated legally to the actual death of the patient by US state legislatures and has been upheld by the courts. Publication of these articles in *JAMA* has had a significant and positive effect on the practice of neurology and on the proper medical and ethical means of deciding the prognosis of the comatose patient in general, and the patient with brain death in particular.

During the past 20 years, PVS and the minimal conscious state have been defined as being separate and identifiable from the comatose state. Positive developments include reports of patients in PVS regaining consciousness within a few weeks. Consciousness may be regained after being in PVS within the first 6 months, although regaining consciousness after 1 year in PVS is infrequent. Additional issues involve recovery of consciousness and recovery of function. The former refers to regaining wakefulness, awareness, and self-awareness. The latter includes meaningful interaction and comprehensiveness with others and the environment, the ability to learn, care for self, and participation in life's activities. Clearly, a meaningful and functional return to consciousness occurs with regularity from PVS and also from the minimal conscious state. It is, therefore, vital for the clinician to observe and recognize a patient's emergence from PVS into the minimal conscious state and to provide maximal clinical support with psychological and physical rehabilitation to allow for the possibility of full consciousness to develop.[1-3,7-8]

Some remarkable advances in the understanding of PVS and the minimal conscious state have occurred recently. Owen et al[9-10] assessed patients with disorders of consciousness, including PVS. For patients who retain motor function, behavioral testing supported by structural imaging and neurophysiological findings can measure accurately the patient's level of wakefulness and self-awareness. However, patients with no motor function can be extremely difficult to evaluate for level of consciousness and their cognitive abilities to perceive and understand commands. Owen et al[9-10] described a novel approach to this conundrum, using functional magnetic resonance imaging to demonstrate preserved conscious awareness in a patient fulfilling the criteria for a diagnosis of being in a vegetative state. Using functional magnetic resonance imaging, the authors showed that supplementary motor area activity during tennis imagery was identical in a patient diagnosed as being in a vegetative state and in a healthy volunteer. Furthermore, activity in the parahippocampal gyrus, posterior parietal lobe, and lateral premotor cortex in a PVS patient and in a healthy volunteer were also identical while imagining moving around a house. Thus, a patient in PVS who appears unaware of the environment and commands actually may be fully aware and cognitively intact but unable to show any response to stimuli. This is a major step forward in understanding the spectrum of PVS and also minimal conscious state cognitive abilities and the ethical and clinical needs to respect the patient's humanity and need for dignified care.

In 2007, Schiff et al[11] reported that a severely brain-injured patient in the minimal conscious state who underwent deep brain stimulation (DBS) showed significant behavioral improvement in attentiveness, recovery of spoken language and oral feeding, and in control of limb movements with central thalamic DBS.[11] This dramatic clinical response has provided a framework for future more comprehensive DBS interventions in a larger number of patients in the minimal conscious state and also PVS. It will be important to map thalamic nuclei to determine the responses to DBS that provide for improved alertness, language functions, and voluntary limb and facial movements. The thalamus is interposed between the brainstem and basal forebrain consciousness arousal systems. It is integrated into a reverberatory, reciprocal oscillatory loop activity with specific neuroanatomical connectivity with a broad representation of cerebral cortex involving multiple cognitive functions.[12-13] As pioneered by Schiff et al,[11] the defining and modulation of the structural and functional substrates of consciousness, of the human mind, of human thinking, and decision making represent a vital and dynamic new field for neuroscience.

In his 1994 book *The Astonishing Hypothesis*,[14] Crick opens with the following: "The Astonishing Hypothesis is that 'You', your joys and your sorrows, your memories and your ambitions, your sense of personal identity and free will, are in fact no more than the behavior of a vast assembly of nerve cells, and their associated molecules. As Lewis Carroll's Alice might have phrased it: 'You're nothing but a pack of neurons.' This hypothesis is so alien to the ideas of most people alive today that it can truly be called astonishing."[14] Crick's point, directly stated, is that there is no separate mind from the brain, the mind is the brain. Cartesian logic of a separate mind and brain is an archaic philosophical concept displaced by current functional magnetic resonance imaging, DBS studies, years of meticulous clinical-neuropathologic studies, and experimental neurophysiological animal studies that have proven that consciousness and mind are embedded into specific neuroanatomical arousal and behavioral circuits. Crick is right that as astonishing as it may be to some, it is now clear that coma, consciousness, and cognition are neural-directed constructs and probably result from mathematical computations yet to be discovered.

Research into the causes of coma and the brain regions involved has moved ahead rapidly in the past 40 years since the publication of the *JAMA* classic article in 1968.[5] The longitudinal course of neurological diseases causal of coma often shows spontaneous improvement, and this is quantified using the neurological examination, imaging studies, clinical chemistries, and electroencephalographic monitoring. The future for therapy of chronic coma, chronic PVS, and the chronic minimal conscious state will require basic studies in neuroregeneration, growth factors, differentiation factors, neurogenesis, and synaptic reinervation. The neuromic program[15] for neuronal and glial differentiation will be essential for reproducing these molecular and structural events first in cell culture, in experimental animals with lesions causal of coma, and then applied to patients who are comatose. Stem cell research in which human adult skin cells are converted into induced pluripotential stem cells, differentiated into neurons or glia, and then differentiated to form neural circuits in vitro will be the first necessary step in bringing the technology of neuroregeneration from the bench to the bedside. These approaches will take time to develop, but they will be achieved and provide the means to treat patients who are comatose.

AUTHOR INFORMATION

Corresponding Author: Roger N. Rosenberg, MD, Department of Neurology and Alzheimer's Disease Center, University of Texas Southwestern Medical Center, 5323 Harry Hines Blvd, Dallas, TX 75390 (roger.rosenberg@utsouthwestern.edu).
Financial Disclosures: None reported. **Author Affiliations:** Department of Neurology and Alzheimer's Disease Center,

11. Sent: Wed, 25 Mar 2009 7:10 am
Subject: Allow assisted suicide, expert on law, health urges Canada

——Original Message——
From: Canadian Physicians for Life <info@physiciansforlife.ca>
To: info@physiciansforlife.ca
http://www.ottawacitizen.com/news/Allow+assisted+suicide+expert+healt h+urges+Canada/1423971/story.html
By Brendan Kennedy, The Ottawa Citizen
March 25, 2009 6:34 AM

OTTAWA-Assisted suicide should be decriminalized in Canada to allow competent and informed people to make decisions about how they die, and because current laws are inconsistent and ineffective, an expert in health law and policy told an Ottawa audience Tuesday night. "My position is grounded in two core ethical values: autonomy and equality," said Jocelyn Downie, Canada Research Chair in health law and policy and professor of law and medicine at Dalhousie University.

Using logical argumentation, Downie made the case that assisted suicide should be decriminalized because individuals already have the right to refuse life-saving medical treatment and to request that such treatment be withdrawn, there is widespread support among the Canadian public for decriminalization, there is no credible evidence to suggest that decriminalizing assisted suicide will lead to higher rates of suicide, vulnerable people can be protected under properly crafted legislation and attempted suicide is not a crime.

"If I'm able-bodied, I can commit suicide. If I'm physically disabled, I cannot ... on equality grounds, this compels us to decriminalize assisted suicide." Downie, author of Dying Justice: A Case for Decriminalizing Euthanasia and Assisted Suicide in Canada, spoke to about 100 people assembled at Nouvelle Scène in Lowertown for "Whose Life is it Anyway? Assisted suicide in Canada," a talk hosted by the Canadian Institutes of Health Research as part of their Café Scientifique discussion series, which aims to engage the public on issues of Canadian health research.

Downie said she had already written a bill that would decriminalize assisted suicide in Canada in order to begin a concrete discussion on the topic, but she said she had no strategy on getting it into parliament. Her proposed bill would require that an individual seeking assisted suicide to be deemed competent by experts, that they make a formal declaration of their decision to seek assisted suicide and that they agree to provide information about themselves to a commission which would monitor cases and report back to parliament. Several audience members, some identifying themselves as members of the pro-life lobby, criticized the format of the event, saying only one side of the debate was represented by an expert.

Discussion moderator Colleen Flood, scientific director of CIHR, said the format was designed to focus on a single Canadian researcher and allow them sufficient time to present their research, and that the counterpoint of the argument would come from the question-and-answer portion. Several audience members, including Conservative MPs Rod Bruinooge and Pierre Lemieux, criticized Downie's position. Bruinooge argued that, if the government were to sanction suicide, it could hinder efforts to dissuade depressed teens from killing themselves. Bruinooge made specific mention of aboriginal youth, who have a much higher rate of suicide than the non-aboriginal population. Downie said that argument could not be sustained because Canadian law already permitted attempted suicide and recognized that suicide could be a rational choice. In an interview after the discussion, Downie said a good death was defined by the individual." It's what the individual determines to be a good death," she said, adding that some people see a good death as one in which you endure pain and others prefer no pain at all. If we fail to confront these difficult questions about death and dying and we fail to demand Canadian legislators to address this issue, "We will all collectively fail in our efforts to truly care for the dying," she said © Copyright (c) The Ottawa Citizen

Doctors face orders to 'kill on demand'New assisted suicide law requires physicians to act May 02, 2009 By Bob Unruh WorldNetDaily
http://wnd.com/index.php?fa=PAGE.view&pageId=96777

Physicians in Montana could be facing "kill-on-demand" orders from patients who want to commit suicide if a district court judge's opinion pending before the state Supreme Court is affirmed. The case has attracted nominal attention nationwide, but lawyers with the Christian Legal Service have filed a friend-of-the-court brief in the pending case because of what it would mean to doctors within the state, as well as the precedent it would set. The concern is over the attack on doctors' ethics and religious beliefs– as well as the Hippocratic oath – that may be violated by a demand that they prescribe deadly chemicals or in some other way assist in a person's death. M. Casey Mattox, a lawyer with the CLS, told WND that states allowing a "right to die" across the country – Oregon and Washington – include an opt-out provision for physicians with ethical or religious opposition to participating in killing a patient. Montana's situation, created late last year in a decision from First District Court Judge Dorothy Mc-

Carter in the Baxter et al. v. Montana case, is different. There is no provision for a doctor to refuse such "treatment" for a patient. Just how did America arrive at a court case ordering doctors to help a suicide? Read it in "The Marketing of Evil: How Radicals, Elitists, and Pseudo-Experts Sell Us Corruption Disguised as Freedom" In that case, Robert Baxter, 75, a retired truck driver from Billings who suffers from lymphocytic leukemia, filed the lawsuit along with four physicians in the state's district court system. They were aided in the case by the assisted suicide advocacy group Compassion & Choices, formerly known as the Hemlock Society. Baxter told the organization's magazine that society already provides death when animals are suffering." I just feel if we can do it for animals," Baxter said, "we can do it for human beings." The CLS, joined by the Christian Medical Association, yesterday filed briefs asking the state Supreme Court to protect the conscience rights of healthcare professionals. The groups, representing more than 18,000 Christian medical and legal professions, are urging the court to reverse the district court's decision and recognize a right not to participate in assisted suicide. "The trial court's decision to create a constitutional right to 'obtain assistance from a medical care provider in the form of obtaining a prescription for lethal drugs' threatens the rights of healthcare professionals and institutions that hold sincere ethical, moral, and religious objections to participating in the intentional killing of their patients," Mattox said.

"Medical professionals should not be coerced to violate the Hippocratic Oath in order to practice in Montana," he said. If a "right to die" is to be recognized, it should be developed from the people through the legislative process, not imposed by a single judge, the brief also argues. The district decision, the groups also point out, would seriously undermine the relationship between doctors and patients. Patients could be uncomfortable knowing their doctor had provided a lethal dose to another patient, and doctors would have concerns about such demands from patients." At a time when states are experiencing a healthcare shortage, making Montana the only state in the union to coerce professionals to assist in suicides could jeopardize the state's healthcare system," Mattox said. He told WND that the effort clearly is part of a nationwide agenda to impose and mandate ethical standards on Americans. Similar are the Obama administration's suggestions that that pharmacists may not have the right to refuse to dispense abortion-inducing medications, and doctors may not have a conscience right to refuse to do abortions, he said." I don't know where it's coming from, but there is certainly a push from government to tell people to set aside religious or ethical qualms and to abide by whatever the government tells you is appropriate," he said Mattox said the state still has several weeks to file its briefs in the Montana case, and then there will be further arguments on behalf of requiring doctors to provide terminal treatment." A mentally competent, terminally ill Montanan should have the right to choose a peaceful death, when confronted by death," Kathryn Tucker, Compassion & Choices director of legal affairs, told KTVQ-TV, Billings. But Montana Assistant Attorney General Anthony Johnston disagrees. Etc, etc....

Euthanasia laws needed (II)

National Post Published: Tuesday, August 04, 2009 Re: We Need Euthanasia Laws, letter to the editor, July 31.Letter-writer Gary Rose contends that "doctor-assisted suicide is theoretically illegal in Canada." That is incorrect: All assisted suicides, including doctor-assisted suicides, are illegal in Canada and punishable by up to 14 years of imprisonment. Prescribing or administering pain-relief treatment that is necessary to relieve pain, and given with a primary intention to achieve that, is not considered euthanasia or assisted suicide, even if it could shorten life (a rare situation). Euthanasia requires a primary intention to kill the patient and assisted suicide a primary intention to help the patient to kill herself or recklessness as to whether she will do so. Ethically and legally valid Do Not Resuscitate orders are not euthanasia or assisted suicide. Neither do "living wills" — refusals of life-prolonging treatment — result in euthanasia. There is an ethical and legal difference between killing someone and allowing them to die naturally of their underlying disease. Moreover, living wills, are legally binding on doctors, not just "a consideration that a doctor weighs when deciding to prolong a life by extraordinary means," as Mr. Rose believes.

The law as it currently stands protects doctors in all these respects and requires doctors to take into account, contrary to Mr. Rose's impression, all aspects of patient suffering, including their needs and wishes concerning life-prolonging treatment. We must be very clear in debating euthanasia and physician-assisted suicide. Otherwise, we might end up legalizing those interventions through confusion, which may sometimes be intentionally generated in order to promote their legalization.

Margaret Somerville, McGill Centre for Medicine, Ethics and Law, Montreal.
http://www.montrealgazette.com/opinion/letters/Words+matter+euthanasia+debate/1853859/story.html

Words matter in euthanasia debate

The Gazette August 2, 2009 Re: "Terminally-ill doctor explains why he prefers to die" (Opinion, July 29)Martin Welsh's deeply thoughtful article concerns refusal of life-prolonging treatment, including artificial hydration and nutrition. In Canada, competent adults have an absolute right to refuse such treatment and through "advance directives" (living wills and durable powers of attorney or mandates) they can ensure that their wishes in this regard are respected should they become incompetent. What those wishes are is a personal moral judgment.

In my article, "Doctors should kill the pain, not the patient" (Gazette, July 28), I explained that, to promote their cause, some pro-euthanasia advocates wrongly label providing pain relief treatment that is necessary to relieve pain, but could shorten life, as euthanasia. The same wrong labelling by euthanasia advocates occurs with refusals of life-prolonging treatment, as described in Welsh's article. When the withdrawal is ethically justified (with informed consent or because it's medically futile - that is, serves no medical purpose) it is not euthanasia. The person is not intentionally killed, but dies a natural death from his or her underlying illness.

Unfortunately, some pro-life advocates also wrongly label all withdrawals of life-prolonging treatment as euthanasia. In doing so, they are risking their position being used to support euthanasia properly so-called. Withdrawals that are not ethically justified - and we may disagree which are and which are not - would be euthanasia; they are intentional killing by omission. But, as explained above, ethically justified withdrawals are not euthanasia.

MargaretSomerville   McGill University
Montreal© Copyright (c) The Montreal Gazette

Already AIDS and other disease epidemics, starvation, exile, war, famine and displacement are depopulating whole nations, to say nothing of the ominous signs in nature and environment on a global scale, that life on our planet is getting distinctly unfriendly, even toxic, much of it a consequence of mankind's heedless, irresponsible greed and mismanagement. Some nations and their leaders are beginning to wake up to the threat that they are no longer reproducing enough children to replace themselves and protect their nations from extinction, but some like Planned Parenthood, are pursuing their abortion agenda with single-minded intensity. When Amnesty International asks its supporting nations to declare abortion a fundamental "right" what do they actually stand for? We also have to wade through the quagmire of child abuse, internationally rampant child pornography, homosexual "marriage," the corruption of research by the pharmaceutical companies and their mega-dollars seducing clinical researchers and distorting results, fraudulent claims, etc...to say nothing of unethical practices in politics, business and virtually all other aspects of life. Yes indeed, doctors and many others have, by these acts, deserved that their souls bear the "mark of Cain, "[Gen 4:15] on them for offending God in these and many other ways. Some are so deeply involved in what they are doing that they have not even considered, or have lost a sense of the rights and wrongs of their behavior; we have lost a sense of sin!

For each physician, medical researcher, nurse etc, and each priest working in a clinical setting, for those that will read and heed this reminder, I believe that I was sent back, partly because I still have much work to do on my own soul, and partly to give this warning to my fellow physicians, that all this behavior which so offends God, and in the way we treat fellow human beings, some of whom happen to become our patients, is bringing His Wrath down upon, not just us, but upon the world. None of those who read this document, whatever they think of it, will be able to say they did not know. <u>It is not my task to make anyone believe; it is my task, and yours, to make fellow physicians aware, and to encourage them to repent and seek God's Mercy.</u>

Were people living the Great Commandments of Love, the myriad of accidents causing some of these strange events of science would not be occurring. By Faith and prayer, God willing,   the women would not be sterile and in need of this peculiar field of medicine to cause them to have a child in spite of their sterility. I give you Sarah,(Gn34:9-15) and Anne,(Hannah in 1Samuel 1:9-28) and Elizabeth(Lk1:5-25); for nothing is impossible to God!(Lk1:38). There appears to be no Faith in the Creator of All present in the medical sciences and, indeed, many of the fields of science today.

Of course, all who believe in God know that there are ALWAYS dire consequences when , in Gods time, He hands out punishment to those who do not repent' but, in 2 Timothy 4: 1-5 Saint Paul tells us; "before God and before Jesus Christ who is to be judge of the living and the dead, I put this duty upon you,(my emphasis) in the name of his Appearing and of his kingdom: proclaim the message and, welcome or unwelcome, insist on it. Refute falsehood, correct error, call to obedience-but do all with patience and with the intention of teaching. The time is sure to come when, far from being content with sound teaching, people will be avid for the latest novelty and collect themselves a whole series of teachers according to their own tastes; and then, instead of listening to the Truth, they will turn to myths. Be careful always to choose the right course; be brave under trials; make the preaching of the Good News your life's work, in thoroughgoing service."

On April 30th, 2000, Pope John Paul canonized St Maria Faustina

Kowalska of The Blessed Sacrament. She was the first saint canonized in the new millennium. On that same day he named that first Sunday after Easter, the Feast of Divine Mercy, just as Jesus requested through St Faustina. In doing so, considering all that He had done to bring the devotion to Divine Mercy through to this point of universal recognition, he earned the title of "the Divine Mercy Pope." In his encyclical "Rich in Mercy, (or Dives in Misericordia), our beloved Holy Father John Paul II, echoed the words which Jesus used when speaking of Mercy to St Faustina, from the Beatitude, "Blessed are the merciful, for they shall receive mercy"[Mt5:7]. **He used this text five times and gave new insight into this beatitude as:**

The Great Commandment of Love in the form of a blessing.
The condition of receiving and revealing mercy.
The synthesis of the whole Gospel.
The call to practice mercy.
Fulfilled in the saints:" come blessed of my Father, receive the Father's blessing of eternal life. [Mt25:34]

We would be hard pressed to answer the question, "In what ways have we not yet defied God?" Yet Jesus said to His disciples; "be merciful as your Father is merciful.[Lk 6;36].

Jesus said to St Faustina, "I have all eternity to punish those."(who do not want to heed His Teaching and Example). In the intervening time, we have God's Mercy. Jesus named her "the Apostle and secretary of Mercy" and said to her;

" Daughter, I need sacrifice lovingly accomplished, because that alone has meaning for Me. Enormous indeed are the debts of the world which are due to Me; pure souls can pay them by their sacrifice, exercising mercy in spirit." [Diary, 1316. Divine Mercy In My Soul].

Jesus was just as strident and forceful as St Paul above, when He said to Faustina,

" My daughter, if I demand through you, that people revere My mercy, you should be the first to distinguish yourself by this confidence in My mercy. I demand from you deeds of mercy, which are to arise out of love for Me. You are to show mercy to your neighbour always and everywhere. You must not shrink from this or try to excuse or absolve yourself from it.

I am giving you three ways of exercising mercy toward your neighbour: the first-by deed, the second,-by word, the third-by prayer. In these three degrees is contained the fullness of mercy, and it is unquestionable proof of love for Me. By this means a soul glorifies and pays reverence to My mercy. Yes, the first Sunday after Easter, is the Feast

of Mercy, but there must also be acts of mercy, and I demand the worship of My mercy through the solemn celebration of the Feast and through the veneration of the Image which is painted. By means of this Image I shall grant many graces to souls. It is to be a reminder of the demands of My mercy, because even the strongest Faith, is to no avail without works. [Diary,742].

I propose one Way back to God, by the One Who is, "The Way, the Truth and The Life,"[Jn 14:6] based on some ideas from Scripture, while it is still a time of Mercy from God. I consider this work an act of mercy from God, toward all my brother and sister physicians. This is not to say that I am excluding any others, but for the purposes of this work I am concentrating on those in my profession. My most urgent priority is to ask you all to step out of your comfort zone, study this article and God-centred Medical Oath, see if or when you might be willing to sign one and hang it in your office or clinic, and share a copy with a fellow physician, encouraging them to consider signing and hanging one likewise.

I know it takes a deep examination of conscience to consider first, to what extent do we, or will we live our lives in accordance with the Great Commandments. Have we reached the place were we can sign this covenant and hang it in our office for all our patients to read and comment or ask questions? Would we be willing or able to extend this invitation to other physicians in my or your own area as a challenge to them to live up to these standards for the salvation of their own souls. Most importantly, our works of mercy must be done in love and in union with God. We are all sinners, never judges.

I am Love and Mercy Itself. When a soul approaches me with trust, I fill it with such an abundance of graces, that it cannot contain them within itself, but radiates them to other souls. [Diary 1074]

NB.[*Scriptural references from* The Jerusalem Bible*; Doubleday-English Translation unless otherwise specified.*]

Ruth Oliver,M.B. Ch.B.,F.R.C.P.(C).
For those interested in the actual "Words" see Some examples page 91.
Book, " Medicine of God " ISBN 978-1-926582-43-6

Complete information see :web address http://www.epistleoflove.org/
Email: info@epistleoflove.org

.

Acknowledgements

Fr J. Soria for reviewing and correcting Scriptural/Religious references.
Those who gave permission to quote their articles:
Dr Dianne Irving, M.A., Ph.D. – in Crisis Magazine: Vol. 19, No. 5 May 2001.
Maurice Vellacott, MP, Conservative – Saskatoon-Wanuskewin
Michelle Poblete editor at USA today,for article by James O'Neil
Robert L. Spitzer, M.D.Professor of Psychiatry Columbia University,
Edward J. Furton, M.A., Ph.D.Ethicist and Director of Publications, The National Catholic Bioethics Center,
Erin Wisdom,http://www.stjoenews.net/news/2009/mar/08/beyond-octomom/,
Michael Goodyear, Assistant Professor, Department of Medicine, Dalhousie ,
Margaret Somerville AM, FRSC, DCL,McGill Centre for Medicine, Ethics and Law, McGill University, Montreal.
Dr Paul Ranalli, Canadian Physicians for Life,
Roger Rosenberg,MD,UTSouthwestern.
John Jalsevac, Assistant Editor, LifeSiteNews.
Janis Murrey Program Manager Journals, CMA Publications Canadian Medical Association ,
Roger Collier ,CMAJ .
Vera Hassner Sharav ALLIANCE FOR HUMAN RESEARCH PROTECTION
Debi Vinnedge,founder, Children of God for Life.
NancyValko,Helen Hitchcock; Women for Faith and Family, St Louis,Missouri.
Six doctors who spent their precious time reading, editing and sharing comments on the content of this booklet; Paul Byrne, Mary Chackalakal, Florence Coleman, Ken Fung, Marie Peeters-Ney and Chris Ryan.

ABSTRACT: given 4th June, 1998.
(A Gift of "Words.").

I am He, your Jesus of Merciful Love, the One who holds the Key to Life and Death. As I look upon My beloved Humanity, I see death and destruction all about. Some think they are doing good, but they do evil; some are just doing evil. Children, as atheism is seemingly controlling the scientific world, many things are occurring which are not pleasing to the Lord your God. Much is anathema and My blessing is not upon much which is occurring now. Many pray for My Kingdom to come upon the Earth now and a period of peace will indeed come shortly. In the interim, there must be a period of cleansing, of purification, of returning to Truth.

I the Lord your God, Am Truth! Invoke the Holy Spirit, and open Scripture. Many indeed know the New Testament. In the Old Testament there is much that is pleasing, and much that is unclean in the eyes of the Lord your God. As I cast My eyes on My beloved Humanity, I behold many who are trying to be gods. I hold the keys of Life and Death. There is a time to be born and a time to die. You play with these very facts of life. You are playing with the very existence of the souls of those you work with, and your own souls! I Myself gift many individuals all over the Earth with healing hands. Many whom you designate as incurable, are cured at the hands of My little faithful ones. My Love is no secret; it is for all mankind. It is I who gift each with the needed intellect according to My Will; yet I bid thee pray the Father of Merciful Love, the Our Father, before you interact with other humans in these solemn matters of Life and Death.

I address you Faithful Missionary in the medical world, and with other of My instruments, I address those whose lifestyles are no longer of Me; who live perilously on the precipice of hell <u>which really exists.</u> At this time I enlighten you, Faithful Missionary, a medical professional, that you might be My instrument, to the other medical professionals. I am asking you to light one candle in the darkness, and leave the rest up to Me; in the power of the Holy Spirit I light up all the darkness !